ESSENTIAL TREMOR

A MEDICAL DICTIONARY, BIBLIOGRAPHY,
AND ANNOTATED RESEARCH GUIDE TO
INTERNET REFERENCES

JAMES N. PARKER, M.D.
AND PHILIP M. PARKER, PH.D., EDITORS

ICON Health Publications
ICON Group International, Inc.
4370 La Jolla Village Drive, 4th Floor
San Diego, CA 92122 USA

Publisher, Health Care: Philip Parker, Ph.D.
Editor(s): James Parker, M.D., Philip Parker, Ph.D.

Publisher's note: The ideas, procedures, and suggestions contained in this book are not intended for the diagnosis or treatment of a health problem. As new medical or scientific information becomes available from academic and clinical research, recommended treatments and drug therapies may undergo changes. The authors, editors, and publisher have attempted to make the information in this book up to date and accurate in accord with accepted standards at the time of publication. The authors, editors, and publisher are not responsible for errors or omissions or for consequences from application of the book, and make no warranty, expressed or implied, in regard to the contents of this book. Any practice described in this book should be applied by the reader in accordance with professional standards of care used in regard to the unique circumstances that may apply in each situation. The reader is advised to always check product information (package inserts) for changes and new information regarding dosage and contraindications before prescribing any drug or pharmacological product. Caution is especially urged when using new or infrequently ordered drugs, herbal remedies, vitamins and supplements, alternative therapies, complementary therapies and medicines, and integrative medical treatments.

Cataloging-in-Publication Data

Parker, James N., 1961-
Parker, Philip M., 1960-

        Essential Tremor: A Medical Dictionary, Bibliography, and Annotated Research Guide to Internet References / James N. Parker and Philip M. Parker, editors
             p.   cm.
        Includes bibliographical references, glossary, and index.
        ISBN: 0-497-00423-2
        1. Essential Tremor-Popular works.   I. Title.

Disclaimer

This publication is not intended to be used for the diagnosis or treatment of a health problem. It is sold with the understanding that the publisher, editors, and authors are not engaging in the rendering of medical, psychological, financial, legal, or other professional services.

References to any entity, product, service, or source of information that may be contained in this publication should not be considered an endorsement, either direct or implied, by the publisher, editors, or authors. ICON Group International, Inc., the editors, and the authors are not responsible for the content of any Web pages or publications referenced in this publication.

Copyright Notice

Acknowledgements

The collective knowledge generated from academic and applied research summarized in various references has been critical in the creation of this book which is best viewed as a comprehensive compilation and collection of information prepared by various official agencies which produce publications on essential tremor. Books in this series draw from various agencies and institutions associated with the United States Department of Health and Human Services, and in particular, the Office of the Secretary of Health and Human Services (OS), the Administration for Children and Families (ACF), the Administration on Aging (AOA), the Agency for Healthcare Research and Quality (AHRQ), the Agency for Toxic Substances and Disease Registry (ATSDR), the Centers for Disease Control and Prevention (CDC), the Food and Drug Administration (FDA), the Healthcare Financing Administration (HCFA), the Health Resources and Services Administration (HRSA), the Indian Health Service (IHS), the institutions of the National Institutes of Health (NIH), the Program Support Center (PSC), and the Substance Abuse and Mental Health Services Administration (SAMHSA). In addition to these sources, information gathered from the National Library of Medicine, the United States Patent Office, the European Union, and their related organizations has been invaluable in the creation of this book. Some of the work represented was financially supported by the Research and Development Committee at INSEAD. This support is gratefully acknowledged. Finally, special thanks are owed to Tiffany Freeman for her excellent editorial support.

About the Editors

James N. Parker, M.D.

Dr. James N. Parker received his Bachelor of Science degree in Psychobiology from the University of California, Riverside and his M.D. from the University of California, San Diego. In addition to authoring numerous research publications, he has lectured at various academic institutions. Dr. Parker is the medical editor for health books by ICON Health Publications.

Philip M. Parker, Ph.D.

Philip M. Parker is the Eli Lilly Chair Professor of Innovation, Business and Society at INSEAD (Fontainebleau, France and Singapore). Dr. Parker has also been Professor at the University of California, San Diego and has taught courses at Harvard University, the Hong Kong University of Science and Technology, the Massachusetts Institute of Technology, Stanford University, and UCLA. Dr. Parker is the associate editor for ICON Health Publications.

About ICON Health Publications

To discover more about ICON Health Publications, simply check with your preferred online booksellers, including Barnes&Noble.com and Amazon.com which currently carry all of our titles. Or, feel free to contact us directly for bulk purchases or institutional discounts:

ICON Group International, Inc.
4370 La Jolla Village Drive, Fourth Floor
San Diego, CA 92122 USA
Fax: 858-546-4341
Web site: **www.icongrouponline.com/health**

Table of Contents

FORWARD

In March 2001, the National Institutes of Health issued the following warning: "The number of Web sites offering health-related resources grows every day. Many sites provide valuable information, while others may have information that is unreliable or misleading."[1] Furthermore, because of the rapid increase in Internet-based information, many hours can be wasted searching, selecting, and printing. Since only the smallest fraction of information dealing with essential tremor is indexed in search engines, such as **www.google.com** or others, a non-systematic approach to Internet research can be not only time consuming, but also incomplete. This book was created for medical professionals, students, and members of the general public who want to know as much as possible about essential tremor, using the most advanced research tools available and spending the least amount of time doing so.

In addition to offering a structured and comprehensive bibliography, the pages that follow will tell you where and how to find reliable information covering virtually all topics related to essential tremor, from the essentials to the most advanced areas of research. Public, academic, government, and peer-reviewed research studies are emphasized. Various abstracts are reproduced to give you some of the latest official information available to date on essential tremor. Abundant guidance is given on how to obtain free-of-charge primary research results via the Internet. **While this book focuses on the field of medicine, when some sources provide access to non-medical information relating to essential tremor, these are noted in the text.**

E-book and electronic versions of this book are fully interactive with each of the Internet sites mentioned (clicking on a hyperlink automatically opens your browser to the site indicated). If you are using the hard copy version of this book, you can access a cited Web site by typing the provided Web address directly into your Internet browser. You may find it useful to refer to synonyms or related terms when accessing these Internet databases. **NOTE:** At the time of publication, the Web addresses were functional. However, some links may fail due to URL address changes, which is a common occurrence on the Internet.

For readers unfamiliar with the Internet, detailed instructions are offered on how to access electronic resources. For readers unfamiliar with medical terminology, a comprehensive glossary is provided. For readers without access to Internet resources, a directory of medical libraries, that have or can locate references cited here, is given. We hope these resources will prove useful to the widest possible audience seeking information on essential tremor.

The Editors

---

[1] From the NIH, National Cancer Institute (NCI): **http://www.cancer.gov/cancerinfo/ten-things-to-know**.

CHAPTER 1. STUDIES ON ESSENTIAL TREMOR

Overview

In this chapter, we will show you how to locate peer-reviewed references and studies on essential tremor.

The Combined Health Information Database

The Combined Health Information Database summarizes studies across numerous federal agencies. To limit your investigation to research studies and essential tremor, you will need to use the advanced search options. First, go to **http://chid.nih.gov/index.html**. From there, select the "Detailed Search" option (or go directly to that page with the following hyperlink: **http://chid.nih.gov/detail/detail.html**). The trick in extracting studies is found in the drop boxes at the bottom of the search page where "You may refine your search by." Select the dates and language you prefer, and the format option "Journal Article." At the top of the search form, select the number of records you would like to see (we recommend 100) and check the box to display "whole records." We recommend that you type "essential tremor" (or synonyms) into the "For these words:" box. Consider using the option "anywhere in record" to make your search as broad as possible. If you want to limit the search to only a particular field, such as the title of the journal, then select this option in the "Search in these fields" drop box. The following is what you can expect from this type of search:

- **Current Understanding and Treatment of Phonatory Disorders in Geriatric Populations**

    Source: Current Opinion in Otolaryngology and Head and Neck Surgery. 8(3): 158-164. June 2000.

    Contact: Available from Lippincott Williams and Wilkins. 12107 Insurance Way, Hagerstown, MD 21740. (800) 637-3030. Fax (301) 824-7390. Website: www.lww.com.

    Summary: Developmental changes from infancy through old age have long been recognized in all systems related to voice reproduction. The increasing numbers of people surviving well into the seventh, eighth, and ninth decades of life demand a thorough understanding of these changes and of the disorders of voice that affect this population. However, research in the treatment of age related voice disorders is in its infancy. This article organizes what is known about multisystem changes, explains the effects those changes may have on phonation, and describes recent treatment approaches to dysphonias (voice disorders or loss of voice) resulting from the aging process and those resulting from diseases prevalent in the geriatric population. The authors discuss age related effects on glottal closure, on vocal fold tension and mass, and on mucosal stiffness, age related glandular changes, firing characteristics of laryngeal muscles in the aged, the effects of aging on motor unit control properties, and psychosocial and other effects of aging. Causes of voice disorders in the geriatric population can include systemic diseases, drug effects, lesions, inflammatory conditions, peripheral nerve involvement, and central neurologic disorders. The authors outline treatment approaches for patients with Parkinson disease, amyotrophic lateral sclerosis (ALS), multiple sclerosis (MS), **essential tremor,** and age related presbyphonia (presbylaryngis). The authors stress that the ability to produce an acceptable voice, which carries communication, is vital to an acceptable quality of life. 2 tables. 40 references.

Federally Funded Research on Essential Tremor

The U.S. Government supports a variety of research studies relating to essential tremor. These studies are tracked by the Office of Extramural Research at the National Institutes of Health.[2] CRISP (Computerized Retrieval of Information on Scientific Projects) is a searchable database of federally funded biomedical research projects conducted at universities, hospitals, and other institutions.

Search the CRISP Web site at **http://crisp.cit.nih.gov/crisp/crisp_query.generate_screen**. You will have the option to perform targeted searches by various criteria, including geography, date, and topics related to essential tremor.

For most of the studies, the agencies reporting into CRISP provide summaries or abstracts. As opposed to clinical trial research using patients, many federally funded studies use animals or simulated models to explore essential tremor. The following is typical of the type of information found when searching the CRISP database for essential tremor:

- **Project Title: CENTRAL RHYTHMOGENESIS AND BEHAVIOR**

  Principal Investigator & Institution: Welsh, John P.; Associate Scientist; None; Oregon Health & Science University Portland, or 972393098

  Timing: Fiscal Year 2002; Project Start 01-MAR-1993; Project End 31-AUG-2007

  Summary: (provided by applicant): This project will focus on the importance of neuronal synchrony and oscillation within the inferior olive, one of the two major afferent systems of the cerebellum. The inferior olive has the highest density of electrotonic synapses and gap junctions in the adult mammalian brain, but their function remains elusive. Our studies will employ a novel genetic tool involving a point-mutation in connexin36 - the protein that assembles neuronal gap junctions - that acts in a dominant-negative manner in vivo to prevent intrinsic connexin36 from assembling gap junctions in dendritic spines of olivary neurons. The basic working hypothesis is

---

[2] Healthcare projects are funded by the National Institutes of Health (NIH), Substance Abuse and Mental Health Services (SAMHSA), Health Resources and Services Administration (HRSA), Food and Drug Administration (FDA), Centers for Disease Control and Prevention (CDCP), Agency for Healthcare Research and Quality (AHRQ), and Office of Assistant Secretary of Health (OASH).

that electrotonic synapses among inferior olivary neurons are fundamental for cerebellar coordination of movement. There are four specific aims. Aim I will determine whether inhibition of connexin36-mediated gap junctions blocks inferior olivary neurons' sub-threshold oscillations in membrane potential and remediates a pathological tremor. Aim 2 will determine how inhibition of connexin36-mediated gap junctions within the inferior olive will alter synchrony and neuronal interaction within cerebellar cortex. Aim 3 will determine whether inhibition of neuronal synchrony within the inferior olive will alter the timing and trajectory of a spatially-guided movement involving a conditioned tongue protrusion behavior. Aim 4 will determine whether blockade of connexin36 mediated gap junctions within the inferior olive will prevent the death of Purkinje cells after brain ischemia. The research will provide fundamental information regarding the role of neuronal synchrony in motor control and for driving Purkinje cells into death after brain ischemia. Moreover, the research is likely to provide a greater understanding of **essential tremor,** which has been associated with pathological inferior olivary oscillation

Website: http://crisp.cit.nih.gov/crisp/Crisp_Query.Generate_Screen

- **Project Title: CLONING OF A GENE FOR PARKINSONISM ON CHROMOSOME 4P**

Principal Investigator & Institution: Hardy, John A.; Professor; Mayo Clinic Coll of Med, Jacksonville Mayo Clinic Jacksonville Jacksonville, Fl 322243899

Timing: Fiscal Year 2002

Summary: We have identified a chromosome 4p haplotype which segregates with L-dopa responsive, Lewy body parkinsonism. The haplotype also co-segregates with a phenotype of **essential tremor** prevalent in the family. Statistical evidence suggests this region is likely to contain the mutant gene responsible for these alternate phenotypes. We have identified two other families (independent datasets) to support our claim. An Italian kindred which shares chromosome 4p markers that segregate with early-onset Parkinson's disease and Family J (Wisconsin) with early onset Parkinson's diseases that strikingly resembles (clinically, Pathologically and geographically) disease in the Iowa kindred. This latter remains to be genetically and genealogically linked but is likely to be an additional branch. Using these resources, and additional families identified by the Clinical and Linkage Cores, our application is to use positional cloning strategies to identify the mutant gene. This will be achieved by the following techniques: (1) further genetic analysis of families putatively linked to chromosome 4p to refine a minimal haplotype (genetic analyses will include heterogeneity testing, multipoint/haplotype analysis of cross-over data and fine mapping using linkage disequilibrium): (2) rapid cDNA candidates gene sequencing from the linked interval; (3) construction and definition of a physical map (minimal framework contig in YACs, redundant tiling path in PACs, STS, STRP and EST localization); (4) gene identification (EST extention using full length cDNA libraries, exon trapping/cDNA selection, intron/exon genomic organisation, expression analysis) followed by gene sequencing in the search for mutation(s) segregating with early onset parkinsonism. Our subsidiary goals are to determine the importance of this locus in other familiar and idiopathic parkinsonian syndromes, in part through collaboration with the Epidemiology and Genetics of Parkinson's Disease Project (P.I. Walter Rocca, Co-PI Dernetriuus Maraganore).

Website: http://crisp.cit.nih.gov/crisp/Crisp_Query.Generate_Screen

- **Project Title: CNS LESIONS EFFECTS ON DRUG ACTION**

  Principal Investigator & Institution: Harvey, John A.; Professor; Pharmacology and Physiology; Drexel University College of Medicine 245 N 15Th St Philadelphia, Pa 19102

  Timing: Fiscal Year 2002; Project Start 01-SEP-1988; Project End 31-MAY-2004

  Summary: (Applicant's Abstract) Our previous research, employing classical conditioning of the rabbit's nictitating membrane response has demonstrated that both associative learning and motor performance are critically dependent on the normal activity of the inferior olivary nucleus. Learning during classical conditioning involves a precise timing mechanism as indicated by its exquisite sensitivity to the temporal parameters of stimulus interval. Our work and that of others suggest that the synchronized oscillatory activity of olivary neurons may provide this timing mechanism. Moreover, serotonin (5-HT) has been demonstrated to regulate the rhythmic activity of the inferior olivary nucleus and also to determine the rate of learning and its motor expression. Both of these actions are mediated by the 5-HT2A receptor. Thus, we have hypothesize that 5-HT agonists and antagonists can increase or decrease the rate of learning and optimum level of motor function by acting at 5-HT2A receptors located on olivary neurons so as to enhance the ability of the olive to coordinate a neural network that determines the efficiency of learning and its motor expression. Experiments will be carried out to produce general or specific 5-HT denervations in order to assess the role of presynaptic 5-HT release on the acquisition of learning and motor performance. Systemic and intracerebral injections of 5-HT2A agonists and antagonists will allow us to identify the critical sites at which normal function can be restored. Other experiments will examine the 5-Ht mechanisms through which tremorogenic agents that act directly on the inferior olive impair learning and performance. Finally, we will examine whether the ability of some 5-HT2A antagonists to retard learning and motor function is due to their actions as inverse agonists. These experiments will provide clues concerning the role of the olivocerebellar system in learning and motor performance and possibly in the treatment of dysfunctions in learning and motor function. For example, 5-HT has been implicated in **essential tremor** and 5-HT2A receptor blockade has been demonstrated to be sufficient for antipsychotic action.

  Website: http://crisp.cit.nih.gov/crisp/Crisp_Query.Generate_Screen

- **Project Title: CORE--NEUROTOXICOLOGY AND NEURODEGENERATIVE DISEASES FACILITY**

  Principal Investigator & Institution: Mayeux, Richard P.; Professor of Neurology, Psychiatry and e; Columbia University Health Sciences Po Box 49 New York, Ny 10032

  Timing: Fiscal Year 2002

  Summary: Research efforts in the Neurotoxicology/Neurodegenerative Disease Research Core will be under the direction of Dr. Richard Mayeux and will span clinical, epidemiological, and mechanistic studies of lead and mercury poisoning and neurodegenerative diseases including Parkinson s and Alzheimer?s disease. It is anticipated that Dr. Mayeux will form task-oriented working groups which will focus on specific problems within areas of interest. Members of the faculty, postdoctoral fellows and doctoral students will meet monthly to discuss topics of ongoing interest in one of the following areas: 1) gene-environment interactions in the neurodegenerative diseases of aging; 2) molecular mechanisms involved in the perturbation of iron metabolism as it relates to Parkinsonism; 3) genetic susceptibility to Parkinson s disease in first-degree relatives of both sporadic and familial cases and the pattern of inheritance; 4) the genetic bases of **essential tremor** and Alzheimer?s disease; 5) effects of lead on cognitive performance and development of children; 6) relationships between occupational exposure to mercury vapor and the risk of tremor, peripheral neuropathy, cerebellar dysfunction and measures of abnormal balance; 7) mercury exposure derived from amalgams in the mouth and possible associations with neurological dysfunction or neuropsychological deficits; 8) caloric intake, body mass index and the risk of neurodegenerative disease; 9) mitochondrial function in normal aging, Parkinson s and Alzheimer s disease; 10) occupational mercury exposure and the risk of memory and visuospatial ability and disturbed mood; 11) molecular mechanisms of lead neurotoxicity; 12) mechanisms of manganese-induced Parkinsonism; and 13) molecular mechanisms of MPTP. Task-oriented working groups will be composed of selected members of the research core, facilities cores and Center staff as needed. The framework in which these work groups will operate will be flexible and will address specific research concentrations dictated by the overall focus of the Center. The specific aims are as follows: 1) to stimulate and guide interdisciplnary research on neurodegenerative diseases; 2) to stimulate and guide research on neurotoxicology with an emphasis on the neurotoxicity of transition and heavy metals; 3) to expand mechanistic and epidemiologic studies among the elderly of Northern Manhattan and; 4) to extend research efforts concerning the interaction of genetic susceptibility markers and environmental exposures in Parkinson?s and Alzheimer?s Disease. It is anticipated that highlights of meetings held in the 12 research areas will be presented at the bi-weekly work-in-progress meetings and that these meetings will provide a vehicle for communication of progress to other members of the Center and outreach programs.

Website: http://crisp.cit.nih.gov/crisp/Crisp_Query.Generate_Screen

- **Project Title: CORE-NEUROTOXICOLOGY/NEURODEGENERATIVE DISEASE RESEARCH**

Principal Investigator & Institution: Graziano, Joseph H.; Professor Public Health And; Columbia Univ New York Morningside 1210 Amsterdam Ave, Mc 2205 New York, Ny 10027

Timing: Fiscal Year 2003; Project Start 01-APR-2003; Project End 31-MAR-2008

Summary: The developing nervous system is vulnerable to adverse effects due to exposures to a variety of substances in the environment, particularly metals and pesticides. At the same time, chronic exposure to low levels of neurotoxicants throughout life can lead to impaired neurologic functioning later in life, particularly in the elderly. As life expectancy increases, and the baby-boom generation approaches retirement age, neurodegenerative diseases such as IPD, **Essential Tremor** and Alzheimer's Disease will have a significant impact on quality of life, and will represent significant financial costs to the health care system. Collectively, the investigators in this research core are interested in understanding the extent to which, and mechanisms 295 whereby, populations exposed to known quantities of neurotoxicants suffer adverse consequences on the nervous system. The populations under investigation, which include birth cohorts in Yugoslavia and northern Manhattan, populations of adults and children chronically exposed to arsenic in drinking water in Bangladesh, and populations of the elderly in northern Manhattan, represent groups of individuals who have been remarkably well characterized for a variety of chemical exposures and other risk factors for adverse neurologic outcomes. At the same time, laboratory based scientists are exploring the mechanisms whereby the compounds of interest alter normal function. The overall goals of the Neurotoxicology/Neurodegenerative Disease Research Core are: I) to promote and facilitate interdisciplinary neuroscience-related research that will define the magnitude of effect of exposure to substances in the environment that are believed to be involved in the etiology of neurologic disease. These substances include metals (Pb, Mn, Fe and As), pesticides (chlorpyrifos, diazinon, propoxur, and others), 13- carboline alkaloids (harmane and harmine), and other factors; and 2) to unravel the cellular and molecular mechanisms whereby these substances exert their effects. The core is responsible for furthering the development of existing and new investigations of environmental exposures that affect the incidence and/or progression of diseases of the central and peripheral nervous systems. The Specific Aims currently under investigation include: 1) to define the cellular and molecular events involved in chemical models of Parkinsonism and in IPD, with the goal of defining those that are common to each; 2) to elucidate the environmental risk factors associated with the onset of IPD, **Essential Tremor,** and Alzheimer's Disease; 3) to examine, in both humans and animal models, the relationship between environmental Pb exposure and brain function, with particular interest in the possible mediating effects of Pb on thyroid hormone fate and transport; 4) to determine whether exposure to arsenic in drinking water is associated with adverse neuropsychologic effects in children, and polyneuropathy in adults; and 5) to develop biomarkers of prenatal pesticide exposure in humans.

Website: http://crisp.cit.nih.gov/crisp/Crisp_Query.Generate_Screen

- **Project Title: GENETICS AND EPIDEMIOLOGY OF ESSENTIAL TREMOR**

Principal Investigator & Institution: Gilbert, John R.; Associate Research Professor; Medicine; Duke University Durham, Nc 27710

Timing: Fiscal Year 2002; Project Start 15-MAR-2002; Project End 28-FEB-2006

Summary: Essential Tremor (ET) is a heterogenous tremor disorder characterized by a core group of features. The tremor syndrome is characterized by postural and kinetic tremor affecting the arms and hands, although the head, voice, and legs may also be affected. Although frequently described as a benign disorder, this is not true; many patients are socially and physically handicapped, with some patients being totally disabled. The differential diagnosis list for ET is extensive including dystonia, Parkinsonism, myoclonus, peripheral neuropathy, and other conditions. Prevalence estimates range widely, depending upon methodology and diagnostic criteria, from 0.003 to as high as 2% in the general population, with as much as 5% of the population affected over the age of 65. There are no known biological or diagnostic neuropathological markers for ET. The estimates of ET cases presenting with a positive family history range from 17.4% to 100%. Recent studies indicate that up to 96% of ET may be dominantly inherited. Clinical and genetic heterogeneity have slowed linkage studies. To date three loci associated with ET have been linked: 1) Familial **Essential Tremor 1** (FET1) has been mapped in a series of Icelandic families on chromosome 3q13; (2) ETM mapped, in four unrelated US families, to chromosome 2p22-p25; and (3) a third locus maps, in a family that segregates both Parkinson's disease and postural tremor consistent with ET, to Chromosome 4p. We have, to date, ascertained, twelve ET and ET/PD linkage quality families. The largest pure ET kindred (DUK13001) have been excluded from known ET loci. The aims of this proposal are to ascertain and sample large families with ET, carry out a complete ET genome scan to establish linkage for these and additional ET families, identify new ET disease loci, and isolate and characterize ET genes, beginning with DUK13001 ET family.

Website: http://crisp.cit.nih.gov/crisp/Crisp_Query.Generate_Screen

- **Project Title: MECHANISM OF DEEP BRAIN STIMULATION**

  Principal Investigator & Institution: Perlmutter, Joel S.; Professor; Radiology; Washington University Lindell and Skinker Blvd St. Louis, Mo 63130

  Timing: Fiscal Year 2002; Project Start 01-APR-2001; Project End 31-MAR-2004

  Summary: (Provided by Applicant): High frequency stimulation of selected brain nuclei has provided dramatic benefit for people with Parkinson disease (PD) and **essential tremor** (ET). Stimulation of the ventral intermediate nucleus (VIM) of the thalamus may abolish contralateral tremor in people with ET or PD. Bilatera" stimulation of the subthalamic nuclei (STN) in people with PD markedly decreases slowness, stiffness, tremor and reduces the need for dopamimetic therapy. Despite these remarkable benefits, the mechanism of action of deep brain stimulation (DES) remains unknown Some investigators have proposed that DBS reduces efferent neuronal firing by either increased inhibition or conduction block. Alternatively, DBS could increase efferent activity, as suggested by our preliminary data and the work of others. We hypothesize that DBS in VIM or STN works by stimulating projection neurons that can be identified by increased blood flow at their terminal fields. We further propose that STN stimulation produces changes in motor behavior or working memory that reflect stimulation of specific brain regions such as supplementary motor area or dorsolateral prefrontal cortex. We plan to use positron emission tomography (PET) to measure blood flow responses to DBS of VIM in ET patients using subtraction image analysis. We will determine whether local blood flow increases or decreases at the sites of the terminal fields of efferent neurons that project from VIM (in ET patients) or STN (in PD patients). We also will vary stimulus variables to produce graded reductions in tremor amplitude and use these different responses to identify regional brain responses that correlate with the clinical effect. In PD patients, we will quantify STN DBS-induced changes in bradykinesia, rigidity, tremor and working memory and correlate them with regional blood flow responses. These studies will permit us to determine whether deep brain stimulation works by driving efferent neurons (cell bodies, axons or both). Further, these investigations will reveal new insights into the mechanisms of how DBS of VIM reduces tremor and how DBS of STN reduces bradykinesia, rigidity, tremor and working memory. Such information may help to optimize treatment with this new modality and potentially suggest alternate approaches to provide additional clinical benefit.

  Website: http://crisp.cit.nih.gov/crisp/Crisp_Query.Generate_Screen

- **Project Title: MOOD EFFECTS OF DEEP BRAIN STIMULATION IN PARKINSONS**

  Principal Investigator & Institution: George, Mark S.; Distinguished Professor; Psychiatry and Behavioral Scis; Medical University of South Carolina P O Box 250854 Charleston, Sc 29425

  Timing: Fiscal Year 2002; Project Start 30-SEP-2000; Project End 31-AUG-2004

  Summary: (Adapted from the Applicant's Abstract): Deep Brain Stimulation (DBS) of the thalamus, globus pallidus (GPi) or subthalamic nucleus (STN) is a new treatment for **essential tremor** and bradykinesia in Parkinson's Disease (PD). The neuropsychological and mood effects of stimulation at these sites are poorly categorized and understood. Major depression (MD) occurs in up to 40% of PD patients. The functional neuroanatomy of normal mood regulation in health and the pathological changes in MD are becoming better understood but still lag behind the neuroanatomical knowledge of motor dysfunction in PD. A key concept developed by the PI and others is that mood is regulated through changes in activity in the anterior paralimbic circuit (APLC) (amygdala, septum, anterior cingulate cortex, anterior temporal poles and orbitofrontal cortex) and that this system functions abnormally in MD. The PI and others have pioneered new treatments for MD JMS, VNS) that have indirectly stimulated this brain circuit. In modem research, no one has used DBS for the primary treatment of MD, although mood effects of DBS have been observed. Based on functional imaging, case report and animal model data, we hypothesize that DBS will cause acute mood changes in PD patients only when DBS affects the APLC. To test this theory that APLC activation is necessary for mood-altering and perhaps antidepressant effects of DBS, we propose to recruit 32 PD patients over a three year period who would fulfill PD clinical indications for DBS (e.g. resistant akinesia, postural rigidity). We will randomly assign these subjects to bilateral DBS at one of two sites either the STN or the GPi. Two days following implantation we will use interleaved DBS/fMRI and intermittently stimulate at the 4 sites on each electrode (bilaterally coordinated), examining changes in self rated mood, psychophysiological measures (HR, BP, GSR, Oxygen saturation), and most importantly, rCBF changes locally and in secondary limbic regions (APLQ. In a masked clinical trial, we will then examine the effects of 4 weeks of a fixed dose of clinically indicated DBS at the implanted site (GPi, STN) on movement, mood and cognition. Subjects with depression symptoms following the 'standard' care will be treated for 4 weeks at the electrode site that on fMRI had the most APLC involvement. The goals of this study are to test this APLC hypothesis of mood regulation and to develop a better working knowledge of the effects of DBS on mood in PD. Thus, we plan to use interleaved fMRI and DBS to directly examine the effects of DBS on hypothesized brain circuits and to correlate this with immediate and longer-term (4 week) behavioral outcomes (mood and cognition).

Website: http://crisp.cit.nih.gov/crisp/Crisp_Query.Generate_Screen

- **Project Title: OPTICAL COHERENCE DOMAIN REFLECTOMETRY IN BRAIN PROBES**

Principal Investigator & Institution: Huang, David; Surgery; Cleveland Clinic Lerner Col/Med-Cwru Cleveland, Oh 44195

Timing: Fiscal Year 2003; Project Start 30-SEP-2003; Project End 31-AUG-2005

Summary: (provided by applicant): The goal of this project is to develop optical coherence domain reflectometry (OCDR) for accurate image guided placement of treatment probes in deep-brain structures. Refined guidance would greatly enhance the effectiveness and safety of deep-brain stimulation (DBS) with implanted electrodes. DBS is an FDA-approved treatment for Parkinson's disease and **essential tremor** that provides long-term relief of symptoms when medications are inadequate. It is also a promising therapy for intractable dystonia, epilepsy, and obsessive-compulsive disorder. Although effective, DBS is not currently a first-line treatment because of difficulties with precise placement, as well as risks of causing hemorrhagic stroke and other complications. Moreover, lengthy intraoperative electrical recordings and stimulus-response observations are currently required to position the probe. An embedded OCDR sensor may provide information on brain structures several millimeters ahead of the probe tip, enabling more precise, rapid, and safe placement. These improvements would allow DBS to benefit more patients. OCDR-guided deep-brain probes could also provide precise delivery of therapeutic vehicles in gene therapy, neurotransplantation, neuro-ablation, and pharmacologic treatments. The investigators include an original developer of OCDR and optical coherence tomography (OCT) in biomedical applications and an expert practitioner and developer of the DBS technique. The combined expertise of this team will take several promising approaches to using

OCDR to identify brain tissue types (cortex, tracts, nuclei, and blood vessels) through a miniature probe. The following Specific Aims are proposed: Aim 1: Develop a combined OCDR/microelectrode brain probe. Aim 2: Distinguish brain tissue types using a dual-wavelength OCDR system that measures tissue reflectivity, attenuation, hydration, and birefringence. Aim 3: Detect blood vessels by Doppler shift and broadening of OCDR spectrum. Aim 4: Develop analysis & display software to identify tissues and guide probe advance. The OCDR brain probe technology will be validated in the laboratory and tested in a rat model. The practical knowledge gained in this pilot project will be used to develop a clinical OCDR-guided deep-brain probe for human DBS studies. Successful completion of this project would greatly benefit patients with many neurologic and psychiatric disorders.

Website: http://crisp.cit.nih.gov/crisp/Crisp_Query.Generate_Screen

- **Project Title: PATHOGENESIS OF ESSENTIAL TREMOR: CEREBELLAR METABOLISM**

Principal Investigator & Institution: Louis, Elan D.; Associate Professor of Neurology; Neurology; Columbia University Health Sciences Po Box 49 New York, Ny 10032

Timing: Fiscal Year 2003; Project Start 01-AUG-2003; Project End 31-JUL-2008

Summary: (provided by applicant): **Essential tremor** (ET) is the most common tremor disorder, twenty times more prevalent than Parkinson's disease. Up to 6% of the general population has ET. Uncontrollable trembling eventually forces 10 - 25% of patients to retire prematurely. There is no cure, and few medications lessen the tremor, although deep brain stimulation has provided promising results. Clinical evidence and neuro-imaging studies suggest that the cerebellum is centrally involved in ET, and evidence from clinical and animal studies suggests that there may be a disturbance in the gamma amino butyric acid (GABA) neurotransmitter system. While ET is clinically progressive, little is known about its underlying pathology. There have been few published postmortem examinations. The fundamental question in ET research is whether an underlying pathology can be identified in terms of morphological or morphometric changes of specific cell types in specific brain regions? Second, is there a neurotransmitter abnormality in ET, either resulting as a consequence of cell loss or in the absence of cell loss? The proposed study will be a collaborative effort involving four centers in the United States and Canada where archival postmortem tissue on 24 ET patients is available. In addition, with the help of the International **Essential Tremor** Foundation, we will establish at Columbia University a centralized repository for new prospectively-collected ET brains, collecting 36 additional ET brains during the five-year period. The 60 ET brains will be compared with 40 control brains. Primary Aim 1 is to study the pathology of ET to determine whether there are changes in specific brain regions. Using conventional morphological methods and quantitative morphometric assessments (stereology), tissue will be examined for changes, including cell loss, in the main region of interest (cerebellar hemispheres) and in secondary regions of interest (red nuclei, thalami, inferior olivary nuclei). We hypothesize that changes and cell loss in the cerebellum will be present to a greater extent in ET than in control brains. Primary Aim 2 is to study the GABA neurotransmitter system. We hypothesize that there will be differences in cerebellar GABA-ergic immuno-labeling in ET compared to control brains. Current therapies for ET have come to us by serendipity and are ineffective in up to 50% of patients. Knowledge of the pathological changes and neurochemical abnormality in ET is critical for the design of new therapies for ET.

Website: http://crisp.cit.nih.gov/crisp/Crisp_Query.Generate_Screen

- **Project Title: POSITIONAL CLONING OF A GENE FOR ESSENTIAL TREMOR**

  Principal Investigator & Institution: Higgins, Joseph J.; Associate Clinical Professor of Pediatri; Mid-Hudson Family Health Institute Suite 101 New Paltz, Ny 12561

  Timing: Fiscal Year 2002; Project Start 01-JAN-2000; Project End 31-DEC-2004

  Summary: Essential tremor (ET), the most common movement disorder in humans, significantly compromises the livelihood or social function of at least 85 percent of the 4 million individuals affected with the disease in the United States. Aggravated by emotions, hunger, fatigue and temperature extremes, the condition may cause a functional disability or even incapacitation. The main clinical feature of ET is postural tremor of the arms, but the head, legs, trunk, voice, jaw, and facial muscles also may be involved. The majority of cases are familial and the disease is usually an autosomal dominant trait with incomplete penetrance. The identification of two susceptibility loci on chromosomes (chr) 2p22-p25 (ETM) and chr 3q13.1 (FET1) implies that ET is genetically heterogeneous. We originally identified the ETM locus in a single American family of Czech descent with pure ET, and later refined the location of the ETM gene to 9.1 centiMorgan region by genotyping three additional families with a similar phenotype. The long-term objectives of the proposal are to identify the other ET susceptibility loci by linkage analysis and to characterize these genes by positional cloning techniques. The specific aims are the following: 1). Collect additional individuals and families with ET. 2). Define the minimal critical region (MCR) that contains ET genes by identifying key recombinants. 3). Construct a high-resolution physical map (contig) of the MCR. 4). Isolate the genes within the contig and evaluate these candidates for disease-causing mutations. The results of this research will enhance our understanding of the human motor system in general and the pathogenesis of tremor in particular. Because current pharmacological treatments for ET have limited efficacy and often become ineffective with advancing disease, identifying the genes that cause ET will facilitate the development of more effective therapeutic strategies.

  Website: http://crisp.cit.nih.gov/crisp/Crisp_Query.Generate_Screen

The National Library of Medicine: PubMed

One of the quickest and most comprehensive ways to find academic studies in both English and other languages is to use PubMed, maintained by the National Library of Medicine.[3] The advantage of PubMed over previously mentioned sources is that it covers a greater number of domestic and foreign references. It is also free to use. If the publisher has a Web site that offers full text of its journals, PubMed will provide links to that site, as well as to sites offering other related data. User registration, a subscription fee, or some other type of fee may be required to access the full text of articles in some journals.

To generate your own bibliography of studies dealing with essential tremor, simply go to the PubMed Web site at **http://www.ncbi.nlm.nih.gov/pubmed**. Type "essential tremor" (or synonyms) into the search box, and click "Go." The following is the type of output you can expect from PubMed for essential tremor (hyperlinks lead to article summaries):

---

[3] PubMed was developed by the National Center for Biotechnology Information (NCBI) at the National Library of Medicine (NLM) at the National Institutes of Health (NIH). The PubMed database was developed in conjunction with publishers of biomedical literature as a search tool for accessing literature citations and linking to full-text journal articles at Web sites of participating publishers. Publishers that participate in PubMed supply NLM with their citations electronically prior to or at the time of publication.

- A case report of complete disappearance of essential tremor after Gamma Knife radiosurgery.
  Author(s): Jawahar A, Cardenas RJ, Zwieg RM, Willis BK, Nanda A.
  Source: J La State Med Soc. 2004 May-June; 156(3): 140-2.
  http://www.ncbi.nlm.nih.gov/entrez/query.fcgi?cmd=Retrieve&db=pubmed&dopt=Abstract&list_uids=15233386

- A comparison of different bedside tests for essential tremor.
  Author(s): Louis ED, Ford B, Wendt KJ, Lee H, Andrews H.
  Source: Movement Disorders : Official Journal of the Movement Disorder Society. 1999 May; 14(3): 462-7.
  http://www.ncbi.nlm.nih.gov/entrez/query.fcgi?cmd=Retrieve&db=pubmed&dopt=Abstract&list_uids=10348470

- A double-blind placebo-controlled trial of topiramate treatment for essential tremor.
  Author(s): Connor GS.
  Source: Neurology. 2002 July 9; 59(1): 132-4.
  http://www.ncbi.nlm.nih.gov/entrez/query.fcgi?cmd=Retrieve&db=pubmed&dopt=Abstract&list_uids=12105323

- A double-blind trial of isoniazid for essential tremor and other action tremors.
  Author(s): Hallett M, Ravits J, Dubinsky RM, Gillespie MM, Moinfar A.
  Source: Movement Disorders : Official Journal of the Movement Disorder Society. 1991; 6(3): 253-6.
  http://www.ncbi.nlm.nih.gov/entrez/query.fcgi?cmd=Retrieve&db=pubmed&dopt=Abstract&list_uids=1681430

- A gene (ETM) for essential tremor maps to chromosome 2p22-p25.
  Author(s): Higgins JJ, Pho LT, Nee LE.
  Source: Movement Disorders : Official Journal of the Movement Disorder Society. 1997 November; 12(6): 859-64.
  http://www.ncbi.nlm.nih.gov/entrez/query.fcgi?cmd=Retrieve&db=pubmed&dopt=Abstract&list_uids=9399207

- A multicenter randomized crossover multiple-dose comparison study of arotinolol and propranolol in essential tremor.
  Author(s): Lee KS, Kim JS, Kim JW, Lee WY, Jeon BS, Kim D.
  Source: Parkinsonism & Related Disorders. 2003 August; 9(6): 341-7.
  http://www.ncbi.nlm.nih.gov/entrez/query.fcgi?cmd=Retrieve&db=pubmed&dopt=Abstract&list_uids=12853233

- A new drug for treatment of essential tremor? Time will tell.
  Author(s): Koller WC.
  Source: Mayo Clinic Proceedings. 1991 October; 66(10): 1085-7.
  http://www.ncbi.nlm.nih.gov/entrez/query.fcgi?cmd=Retrieve&db=pubmed&dopt=Abstract&list_uids=1921492

- **A new twist for stopping the shakes? Revisiting GABAergic therapy for essential tremor.**
  Author(s): Louis ED.
  Source: Archives of Neurology. 1999 July; 56(7): 807-8. Review.
  http://www.ncbi.nlm.nih.gov/entrez/query.fcgi?cmd=Retrieve&db=pubmed&dopt=Abstract&list_uids=10404981

- **A positron emission tomography study of essential tremor: evidence for overactivity of cerebellar connections.**
  Author(s): Jenkins IH, Bain PG, Colebatch JG, Thompson PD, Findley LJ, Frackowiak RS, Marsden CD, Brooks DJ.
  Source: Annals of Neurology. 1993 July; 34(1): 82-90.
  http://www.ncbi.nlm.nih.gov/entrez/query.fcgi?cmd=Retrieve&db=pubmed&dopt=Abstract&list_uids=8517685

- **A preliminary look at the percentage of patients with Restless Legs Syndrome who also have Parkinson Disease, Essential Tremor or Tourette Syndrome in a single practice.**
  Author(s): Walters AS, LeBrocq C, Passi V, Patel S, Hanna PA, Cohen B, Wagner M.
  Source: Journal of Sleep Research. 2003 December; 12(4): 343-5. Review.
  http://www.ncbi.nlm.nih.gov/entrez/query.fcgi?cmd=Retrieve&db=pubmed&dopt=Abstract&list_uids=14633247

- **A randomized placebo-controlled comparative trial of gabapentin and propranolol in essential tremor.**
  Author(s): Gironell A, Kulisevsky J, Barbanoj M, Lopez-Villegas D, Hernandez G, Pascual-Sedano B.
  Source: Archives of Neurology. 1999 April; 56(4): 475-80.
  http://www.ncbi.nlm.nih.gov/entrez/query.fcgi?cmd=Retrieve&db=pubmed&dopt=Abstract&list_uids=10199338

- **A single family with writer's cramp, essential tremor, and primary writing tremor.**
  Author(s): Cohen LG, Hallett M, Sudarsky L.
  Source: Movement Disorders : Official Journal of the Movement Disorder Society. 1987; 2(2): 109-16. Erratum In: Mov Disord 1987; 2(3): 224.
  http://www.ncbi.nlm.nih.gov/entrez/query.fcgi?cmd=Retrieve&db=pubmed&dopt=Abstract&list_uids=3504263

- **A study of hereditary essential tremor.**
  Author(s): Bain PG, Findley LJ, Thompson PD, Gresty MA, Rothwell JC, Harding AE, Marsden CD.
  Source: Brain; a Journal of Neurology. 1994 August; 117 (Pt 4): 805-24.
  http://www.ncbi.nlm.nih.gov/entrez/query.fcgi?cmd=Retrieve&db=pubmed&dopt=Abstract&list_uids=7922467

- **A teaching videotape for the assessment of essential tremor.**
  Author(s): Louis ED, Barnes L, Wendt KJ, Ford B, Sangiorgio M, Tabbal S, Lewis L, Kaufmann P, Moskowitz C, Comella CL, Goetz CC, Lang AE.
  Source: Movement Disorders : Official Journal of the Movement Disorder Society. 2001 January; 16(1): 89-93.
  http://www.ncbi.nlm.nih.gov/entrez/query.fcgi?cmd=Retrieve&db=pubmed&dopt=Abstract&list_uids=11215599

- **Abnormal gating of somatosensory inputs in essential tremor.**
  Author(s): Restuccia D, Valeriani M, Barba C, Le Pera D, Bentivoglio A, Albanese A, Rubino M, Tonali P.
  Source: Clinical Neurophysiology : Official Journal of the International Federation of Clinical Neurophysiology. 2003 January; 114(1): 120-9.
  http://www.ncbi.nlm.nih.gov/entrez/query.fcgi?cmd=Retrieve&db=pubmed&dopt=Abstract&list_uids=12495772

- **Accuracy of reported family histories of essential tremor.**
  Author(s): Busenbark K, Barnes P, Lyons K, Ince D, Villagra F, Koller WC.
  Source: Neurology. 1996 July; 47(1): 264-5.
  http://www.ncbi.nlm.nih.gov/entrez/query.fcgi?cmd=Retrieve&db=pubmed&dopt=Abstract&list_uids=8710092

- **Acoustic voice analysis in patients with essential tremor.**
  Author(s): Gamboa J, Jimenez-Jimenez FJ, Nieto A, Cobeta I, Vegas A, Orti-Pareja M, Gasalla T, Molina JA, Garcia-Albea E.
  Source: Journal of Voice : Official Journal of the Voice Foundation. 1998 December; 12(4): 444-52.
  http://www.ncbi.nlm.nih.gov/entrez/query.fcgi?cmd=Retrieve&db=pubmed&dopt=Abstract&list_uids=9988031

- **Activation mapping in essential tremor with functional magnetic resonance imaging.**
  Author(s): Bucher SF, Seelos KC, Dodel RC, Reiser M, Oertel WH.
  Source: Annals of Neurology. 1997 January; 41(1): 32-40. Erratum In: Ann Neurol 1998 March; 43(3): 410.
  http://www.ncbi.nlm.nih.gov/entrez/query.fcgi?cmd=Retrieve&db=pubmed&dopt=Abstract&list_uids=9005863

- **Acute and chronic effects of clozapine in essential tremor.**
  Author(s): Ceravolo R, Salvetti S, Piccini P, Lucetti C, Gambaccini G, Bonuccelli U.
  Source: Movement Disorders : Official Journal of the Movement Disorder Society. 1999 May; 14(3): 468-72.
  http://www.ncbi.nlm.nih.gov/entrez/query.fcgi?cmd=Retrieve&db=pubmed&dopt=Abstract&list_uids=10348471

- **Acute and chronic effects of propranolol and primidone in essential tremor.**
  Author(s): Koller WC, Vetere-Overfield B.
  Source: Neurology. 1989 December; 39(12): 1587-8.
  http://www.ncbi.nlm.nih.gov/entrez/query.fcgi?cmd=Retrieve&db=pubmed&dopt=Abstract&list_uids=2586774

- **Adrenergic beta 2-selective blocker in isoprenaline-enhanced essential tremor.**
  Author(s): Teravainen H, Huttunen J.
  Source: Movement Disorders : Official Journal of the Movement Disorder Society. 1987; 2(2): 103-8.
  http://www.ncbi.nlm.nih.gov/entrez/query.fcgi?cmd=Retrieve&db=pubmed&dopt=Abstract&list_uids=3332807

- **Agreement among movement disorder specialists on the clinical diagnosis of essential tremor.**
  Author(s): Chouinard S, Louis ED, Fahn S.
  Source: Movement Disorders : Official Journal of the Movement Disorder Society. 1997 November; 12(6): 973-6.
  http://www.ncbi.nlm.nih.gov/entrez/query.fcgi?cmd=Retrieve&db=pubmed&dopt=Abstract&list_uids=9399223

- **Aminophylline and essential tremor.**
  Author(s): Mally J.
  Source: British Journal of Clinical Pharmacology. 1997 October; 44(4): 412.
  http://www.ncbi.nlm.nih.gov/entrez/query.fcgi?cmd=Retrieve&db=pubmed&dopt=Abstract&list_uids=9354319

- **Aminophylline and essential tremor.**
  Author(s): Mally J.
  Source: Lancet. 1989 July 29; 2(8657): 278-9.
  http://www.ncbi.nlm.nih.gov/entrez/query.fcgi?cmd=Retrieve&db=pubmed&dopt=Abstract&list_uids=2569084

- **Anticipation of onset age in hereditary essential tremor.**
  Author(s): Bragoni M, Fabbrini G, Di Legge S, Altieri M, Di Piero V.
  Source: Italian Journal of Neurological Sciences. 1997 February; 18(1): 45-7.
  http://www.ncbi.nlm.nih.gov/entrez/query.fcgi?cmd=Retrieve&db=pubmed&dopt=Abstract&list_uids=9115044

- **Arm tremor in cervical dystonia differs from essential tremor and can be classified by onset age and spread of symptoms.**
  Author(s): Munchau A, Schrag A, Chuang C, MacKinnon CD, Bhatia KP, Quinn NP, Rothwell JC.
  Source: Brain; a Journal of Neurology. 2001 September; 124(Pt 9): 1765-76.
  http://www.ncbi.nlm.nih.gov/entrez/query.fcgi?cmd=Retrieve&db=pubmed&dopt=Abstract&list_uids=11522579

- **Arylsulphatase A (ASA) activity in parkinsonism and symptomatic essential tremor.**
  Author(s): Martinelli P, Ippoliti M, Montanari M, Martinelli A, Mochi M, Giuliani S, Sangiorgi S.
  Source: Acta Neurologica Scandinavica. 1994 March; 89(3): 171-4.
  http://www.ncbi.nlm.nih.gov/entrez/query.fcgi?cmd=Retrieve&db=pubmed&dopt=Abstract&list_uids=7913281

- **Assessing the impact of essential tremor on upper limb function.**
  Author(s): Bain PG, Mally J, Gresty M, Findley LJ.
  Source: Journal of Neurology. 1993 November; 241(1): 54-61.
  http://www.ncbi.nlm.nih.gov/entrez/query.fcgi?cmd=Retrieve&db=pubmed&dopt=Abstract&list_uids=8138823

- **Association between essential tremor and blood lead concentration.**
  Author(s): Louis ED, Jurewicz EC, Applegate L, Factor-Litvak P, Parides M, Andrews L, Slavkovich V, Graziano JH, Carroll S, Todd A.
  Source: Environmental Health Perspectives. 2003 November; 111(14): 1707-11.
  http://www.ncbi.nlm.nih.gov/entrez/query.fcgi?cmd=Retrieve&db=pubmed&dopt=Abstract&list_uids=14594619

- **Attenuation of response to mental stress in patients with essential tremor treated with metoprolol.**
  Author(s): Gengo FM, Kalonaros GC, McHugh WB.
  Source: Archives of Neurology. 1986 July; 43(7): 687-9.
  http://www.ncbi.nlm.nih.gov/entrez/query.fcgi?cmd=Retrieve&db=pubmed&dopt=Abstract&list_uids=3729747

- **Basic mechanisms of action of drugs used in the treatment of essential tremor.**
  Author(s): Guan XM, Peroutka SJ.
  Source: Clinical Neuropharmacology. 1990 June; 13(3): 210-23. Review.
  http://www.ncbi.nlm.nih.gov/entrez/query.fcgi?cmd=Retrieve&db=pubmed&dopt=Abstract&list_uids=1972653

- **Benefits and risks of pharmacological treatments for essential tremor.**
  Author(s): Lyons KE, Pahwa R, Comella CL, Eisa MS, Elble RJ, Fahn S, Jankovic J, Juncos JL, Koller WC, Ondo WG, Sethi KD, Stern MB, Tanner CM, Tintner R, Watts RL.
  Source: Drug Safety : an International Journal of Medical Toxicology and Drug Experience. 2003; 26(7): 461-81. Review.
  http://www.ncbi.nlm.nih.gov/entrez/query.fcgi?cmd=Retrieve&db=pubmed&dopt=Abstract&list_uids=12735785

- **Benign essential tremor in childhood: Symptoms, pathogenesis, treatment.**
  Author(s): Paulson GW.
  Source: Clinical Pediatrics. 1976 January; 15(1): 67-70.
  http://www.ncbi.nlm.nih.gov/entrez/query.fcgi?cmd=Retrieve&db=pubmed&dopt=Abstract&list_uids=1245084

- **Benign essential tremor. A clinical survey of 82 patients from Campania, a region of southern Italy.**
  Author(s): Mengano A, Di Maio L, Maggio MA, Squitieri F, Di Donato M, Barbieri F, Campanella G.
  Source: Acta Neurol (Napoli). 1989 August; 11(4): 239-46.
  http://www.ncbi.nlm.nih.gov/entrez/query.fcgi?cmd=Retrieve&db=pubmed&dopt=Abstract&list_uids=2801257

- **Benign essential tremor: features that aid in diagnosis.**
  Author(s): Paulson GW.
  Source: Postgraduate Medicine. 1982 January; 71(1): 105-7.
  http://www.ncbi.nlm.nih.gov/entrez/query.fcgi?cmd=Retrieve&db=pubmed&dopt=A
  bstract&list_uids=7054770

- **Beta 1 versus nonselective blockade in therapy of essential tremor.**
  Author(s): Larsen TA, Teravainen H.
  Source: Adv Neurol. 1983; 37: 247-51.
  http://www.ncbi.nlm.nih.gov/entrez/query.fcgi?cmd=Retrieve&db=pubmed&dopt=A
  bstract&list_uids=6344590

- **Beta-adrenergic blockers in benign essential tremor.**
  Author(s): Scopa J, Longley BP, Foster JB.
  Source: Curr Ther Res Clin Exp. 1973 February; 15(2): 48-51. No Abstract Available.
  http://www.ncbi.nlm.nih.gov/entrez/query.fcgi?cmd=Retrieve&db=pubmed&dopt=A
  bstract&list_uids=4144219

- **Beta-adrenergic mechanisms in essential tremor.**
  Author(s): Young RR, Shahani BT, Growdon JH.
  Source: Trans Am Neurol Assoc. 1974; 99: 265-7. No Abstract Available.
  http://www.ncbi.nlm.nih.gov/entrez/query.fcgi?cmd=Retrieve&db=pubmed&dopt=A
  bstract&list_uids=4463556

- **beta-Adrenoceptor antagonists and essential tremor.**
  Author(s): Leigh PN, Marsden CD, Twomey A, Jefferson D.
  Source: Lancet. 1981 May 16; 1(8229): 1106.
  http://www.ncbi.nlm.nih.gov/entrez/query.fcgi?cmd=Retrieve&db=pubmed&dopt=A
  bstract&list_uids=6112475

- **beta-Adrenoreceptor antagonists in essential tremor.**
  Author(s): Jefferson D, Jenner P, Marsden CD.
  Source: Journal of Neurology, Neurosurgery, and Psychiatry. 1979 October; 42(10): 904-9.
  http://www.ncbi.nlm.nih.gov/entrez/query.fcgi?cmd=Retrieve&db=pubmed&dopt=A
  bstract&list_uids=512665

- **Beta-adrenoreceptor mechanisms in essential tremor: a comparative single dose study of the effect of a non-selective and a beta-2 selective adrenoreceptor antagonist.**
  Author(s): Cleeves L, Findley LJ.
  Source: Journal of Neurology, Neurosurgery, and Psychiatry. 1984 September; 47(9): 976-82.
  http://www.ncbi.nlm.nih.gov/entrez/query.fcgi?cmd=Retrieve&db=pubmed&dopt=A
  bstract&list_uids=6148382

- **Beta-adrenoreceptor mechanisms in essential tremor; a double-blind placebo controlled trial of metoprolol, sotalol and atenolol.**
  Author(s): Leigh PN, Jefferson D, Twomey A, Marsden CD.
  Source: Journal of Neurology, Neurosurgery, and Psychiatry. 1983 August; 46(8): 710-5.
  http://www.ncbi.nlm.nih.gov/entrez/query.fcgi?cmd=Retrieve&db=pubmed&dopt=Abstract&list_uids=6310053

- **Beta-blockers in essential tremor.**
  Author(s): Larsen TA, Teravainen H.
  Source: Lancet. 1981 September 5; 2(8245): 533.
  http://www.ncbi.nlm.nih.gov/entrez/query.fcgi?cmd=Retrieve&db=pubmed&dopt=Abstract&list_uids=6115285

- **Beta-blockers in isoproterenol-enhanced essential tremor.**
  Author(s): Teravainen H.
  Source: Acta Neurologica Scandinavica. 1984 February; 69(2): 125-7.
  http://www.ncbi.nlm.nih.gov/entrez/query.fcgi?cmd=Retrieve&db=pubmed&dopt=Abstract&list_uids=6143467

- **Bilateral thalamic stimulation for the treatment of essential tremor.**
  Author(s): Pahwa R, Lyons KL, Wilkinson SB, Carpenter MA, Troster AI, Searl JP, Overman J, Pickering S, Koller WC.
  Source: Neurology. 1999 October 22; 53(7): 1447-50.
  http://www.ncbi.nlm.nih.gov/entrez/query.fcgi?cmd=Retrieve&db=pubmed&dopt=Abstract&list_uids=10534249

- **Body mass index in essential tremor.**
  Author(s): Louis ED, Marder K, Jurewicz EC, Watner D, Levy G, Mejia-Santana H.
  Source: Archives of Neurology. 2002 August; 59(8): 1273-7.
  http://www.ncbi.nlm.nih.gov/entrez/query.fcgi?cmd=Retrieve&db=pubmed&dopt=Abstract&list_uids=12164723

- **Botulinum toxin for essential tremor of the voice with multiple anatomical sites of tremor: a crossover design study of unilateral versus bilateral injection.**
  Author(s): Warrick P, Dromey C, Irish JC, Durkin L, Pakiam A, Lang A.
  Source: The Laryngoscope. 2000 August; 110(8): 1366-74.
  http://www.ncbi.nlm.nih.gov/entrez/query.fcgi?cmd=Retrieve&db=pubmed&dopt=Abstract&list_uids=10942143

- **Botulinum toxin restores presynaptic inhibition of group Ia afferents in patients with essential tremor.**
  Author(s): Modugno N, Priori A, Berardelli A, Vacca L, Mercuri B, Manfredi M.
  Source: Muscle & Nerve. 1998 December; 21(12): 1701-5.
  http://www.ncbi.nlm.nih.gov/entrez/query.fcgi?cmd=Retrieve&db=pubmed&dopt=Abstract&list_uids=9843072

- **Botulinum toxin treatment for functional disability induced by essential tremor.**
  Author(s): Pacchetti C, Mancini F, Bulgheroni M, Zangaglia R, Cristina S, Sandrini G, Nappi G.
  Source: Neurological Sciences : Official Journal of the Italian Neurological Society and of the Italian Society of Clinical Neurophysiology. 2000 December; 21(6): 349-53.
  http://www.ncbi.nlm.nih.gov/entrez/query.fcgi?cmd=Retrieve&db=pubmed&dopt=Abstract&list_uids=11441571

- **Characteristics of social phobia among persons with essential tremor.**
  Author(s): Schneier FR, Barnes LF, Albert SM, Louis ED.
  Source: The Journal of Clinical Psychiatry. 2001 May; 62(5): 367-72.
  http://www.ncbi.nlm.nih.gov/entrez/query.fcgi?cmd=Retrieve&db=pubmed&dopt=Abstract&list_uids=11411820

- **Clinical and electromyographic assessment of essential tremor treatment.**
  Author(s): Milanov I.
  Source: Parkinsonism & Related Disorders. 2002 June; 8(5): 343-8.
  http://www.ncbi.nlm.nih.gov/entrez/query.fcgi?cmd=Retrieve&db=pubmed&dopt=Abstract&list_uids=15177063

- **Clinical and electromyographic examinations of patients with essential tremor.**
  Author(s): Milanov I.
  Source: The Canadian Journal of Neurological Sciences. Le Journal Canadien Des Sciences Neurologiques. 2000 February; 27(1): 65-70.
  http://www.ncbi.nlm.nih.gov/entrez/query.fcgi?cmd=Retrieve&db=pubmed&dopt=Abstract&list_uids=10676591

- **Clinical and genetic study of essential tremor in the Italian population.**
  Author(s): Abbruzzese G, Pigullo S, Di Maria E, Martinelli P, Barone P, Marchese R, Scaglione C, Assini A, Lucetti C, Berardelli A, Calzetti S, Bellone E, Ajmar F, Mandich P.
  Source: Neurological Sciences : Official Journal of the Italian Neurological Society and of the Italian Society of Clinical Neurophysiology. 2001 February; 22(1): 39-40.
  http://www.ncbi.nlm.nih.gov/entrez/query.fcgi?cmd=Retrieve&db=pubmed&dopt=Abstract&list_uids=11487191

- **Clinical and genetic study of familial essential tremor in an isolate of Northern Tajikistan.**
  Author(s): Illarioshkin SN, Ivanova-Smolenskaya IA, Rahmonov RA, Markova ED, Stevanin G, Brice A.
  Source: Movement Disorders : Official Journal of the Movement Disorder Society. 2000 September; 15(5): 1020-3.
  http://www.ncbi.nlm.nih.gov/entrez/query.fcgi?cmd=Retrieve&db=pubmed&dopt=Abstract&list_uids=11009220

- **Clinical characteristics of essential tremor: data from a community-based study.**
  Author(s): Louis ED, Ford B, Wendt KJ, Cameron G.
  Source: Movement Disorders : Official Journal of the Movement Disorder Society. 1998 September; 13(5): 803-8.
  http://www.ncbi.nlm.nih.gov/entrez/query.fcgi?cmd=Retrieve&db=pubmed&dopt=Abstract&list_uids=9756149

- **Clinical expression of essential tremor: effects of gender and age.**
  Author(s): Hubble JP, Busenbark KL, Pahwa R, Lyons K, Koller WC.
  Source: Movement Disorders : Official Journal of the Movement Disorder Society. 1997 November; 12(6): 969-72.
  http://www.ncbi.nlm.nih.gov/entrez/query.fcgi?cmd=Retrieve&db=pubmed&dopt=Abstract&list_uids=9399222

- **Clinical features, assessment and treatment of essential tremor.**
  Author(s): Panicker JN, Pal PK.
  Source: J Assoc Physicians India. 2003 March; 51: 276-9. Review.
  http://www.ncbi.nlm.nih.gov/entrez/query.fcgi?cmd=Retrieve&db=pubmed&dopt=Abstract&list_uids=12839351

- **Clinical practice. Essential tremor.**
  Author(s): Louis ED.
  Source: The New England Journal of Medicine. 2001 September 20; 345(12): 887-91. Review.
  http://www.ncbi.nlm.nih.gov/entrez/query.fcgi?cmd=Retrieve&db=pubmed&dopt=Abstract&list_uids=11565522

- **Clinical subtypes of essential tremor.**
  Author(s): Louis ED, Ford B, Barnes LF.
  Source: Archives of Neurology. 2000 August; 57(8): 1194-8.
  http://www.ncbi.nlm.nih.gov/entrez/query.fcgi?cmd=Retrieve&db=pubmed&dopt=Abstract&list_uids=10927801

- **Clinical-molecular study of a family with essential tremor, late onset seizures and periodic paralysis.**
  Author(s): Dominguez-Moran JA, Baron M, de Blas G, Orensanz LM, Jimenez-Escrig A.
  Source: Seizure : the Journal of the British Epilepsy Association. 2000 October; 9(7): 493-7.
  http://www.ncbi.nlm.nih.gov/entrez/query.fcgi?cmd=Retrieve&db=pubmed&dopt=Abstract&list_uids=11034874

- **Cognitive deficits in patients with essential tremor.**
  Author(s): Duane DD, Vermilion KJ.
  Source: Neurology. 2002 June 11; 58(11): 1706; Author Reply 1706.
  http://www.ncbi.nlm.nih.gov/entrez/query.fcgi?cmd=Retrieve&db=pubmed&dopt=Abstract&list_uids=12058116

- **Cognitive deficits in patients with essential tremor.**
  Author(s): Lombardi WJ, Woolston DJ, Roberts JW, Gross RE.
  Source: Neurology. 2001 September 11; 57(5): 785-90.
  http://www.ncbi.nlm.nih.gov/entrez/query.fcgi?cmd=Retrieve&db=pubmed&dopt=Abstract&list_uids=11552004

- **Cognitive functioning in individuals with "benign" essential tremor.**
  Author(s): Lacritz LH, Dewey R Jr, Giller C, Cullum CM.
  Source: Journal of the International Neuropsychological Society : Jins. 2002 January; 8(1): 125-9.
  http://www.ncbi.nlm.nih.gov/entrez/query.fcgi?cmd=Retrieve&db=pubmed&dopt=Abstract&list_uids=11843070

- **Coherence between low-frequency activation of the motor cortex and tremor in patients with essential tremor.**
  Author(s): Halliday DM, Conway BA, Farmer SF, Shahani U, Russell AJ, Rosenberg JR.
  Source: Lancet. 2000 April 1; 355(9210): 1149-53.
  http://www.ncbi.nlm.nih.gov/entrez/query.fcgi?cmd=Retrieve&db=pubmed&dopt=Abstract&list_uids=10791378

- **Community-based data on associations of disease duration and age with severity of essential tremor: implications for disease pathophysiology.**
  Author(s): Louis ED, Jurewicz EC, Watner D.
  Source: Movement Disorders : Official Journal of the Movement Disorder Society. 2003 January; 18(1): 90-3.
  http://www.ncbi.nlm.nih.gov/entrez/query.fcgi?cmd=Retrieve&db=pubmed&dopt=Abstract&list_uids=12518305

- **Comparison of clinical vs. electrophysiological methods of diagnosing of essential tremor.**
  Author(s): Louis ED, Pullman SL.
  Source: Movement Disorders : Official Journal of the Movement Disorder Society. 2001 July; 16(4): 668-73.
  http://www.ncbi.nlm.nih.gov/entrez/query.fcgi?cmd=Retrieve&db=pubmed&dopt=Abstract&list_uids=11481690

- **Comparison of thalamotomy to deep brain stimulation of the thalamus in essential tremor.**
  Author(s): Pahwa R, Lyons KE, Wilkinson SB, Troster AI, Overman J, Kieltyka J, Koller WC.
  Source: Movement Disorders : Official Journal of the Movement Disorder Society. 2001 January; 16(1): 140-3.
  http://www.ncbi.nlm.nih.gov/entrez/query.fcgi?cmd=Retrieve&db=pubmed&dopt=Abstract&list_uids=11215575

- **Contralateral voluntary hand movement inhibits human parkinsonian tremor and variably influences essential tremor.**
  Author(s): Tamas G, Palvolgyi L, Takats A, Szirmai I, Kamondi A.
  Source: Neuroscience Letters. 2004 March 11; 357(3): 187-90.
  http://www.ncbi.nlm.nih.gov/entrez/query.fcgi?cmd=Retrieve&db=pubmed&dopt=Abstract&list_uids=15003281

- Co-occurrence of essential tremor and Parkinson's disease: clinical study of a large kindred with autopsy findings.
  Author(s): Yahr MD, Orosz D, Purohit DP.
  Source: Parkinsonism & Related Disorders. 2003 March; 9(4): 225-31.
  http://www.ncbi.nlm.nih.gov/entrez/query.fcgi?cmd=Retrieve&db=pubmed&dopt=Abstract&list_uids=12618058

- Correlates of functional disability in essential tremor.
  Author(s): Louis ED, Barnes L, Albert SM, Cote L, Schneier FR, Pullman SL, Yu Q.
  Source: Movement Disorders : Official Journal of the Movement Disorder Society. 2001 September; 16(5): 914-20.
  http://www.ncbi.nlm.nih.gov/entrez/query.fcgi?cmd=Retrieve&db=pubmed&dopt=Abstract&list_uids=11746622

- Cortical excitability in patients with essential tremor.
  Author(s): Romeo S, Berardelli A, Pedace F, Inghilleri M, Giovannelli M, Manfredi M.
  Source: Muscle & Nerve. 1998 October; 21(10): 1304-8.
  http://www.ncbi.nlm.nih.gov/entrez/query.fcgi?cmd=Retrieve&db=pubmed&dopt=Abstract&list_uids=9736059

- Cortical silent period in essential tremor.
  Author(s): Shukla G, Bhatia M, Pandey RM, Behari M.
  Source: Electromyogr Clin Neurophysiol. 2003 September; 43(6): 329-33.
  http://www.ncbi.nlm.nih.gov/entrez/query.fcgi?cmd=Retrieve&db=pubmed&dopt=Abstract&list_uids=14535045

- Cortico-cortical inhibition of the motor cortical area projecting to sternocleidomastoid muscle in normals and patients with spasmodic torticollis or essential tremor.
  Author(s): Hanajima R, Ugawa Y, Terao Y, Sakai K, Furubayashi T, Machii K, Uesugi H, Mochizuki H, Kanazawa I.
  Source: Electroencephalography and Clinical Neurophysiology. 1998 October; 109(5): 391-6.
  http://www.ncbi.nlm.nih.gov/entrez/query.fcgi?cmd=Retrieve&db=pubmed&dopt=Abstract&list_uids=9851295

- Criteria for the diagnosis of essential tremor.
  Author(s): Bain P, Brin M, Deuschl G, Elble R, Jankovic J, Findley L, Koller WC, Pahwa R.
  Source: Neurology. 2000; 54(11 Suppl 4): S7.
  http://www.ncbi.nlm.nih.gov/entrez/query.fcgi?cmd=Retrieve&db=pubmed&dopt=Abstract&list_uids=10854345

- Deep brain stimulation for essential tremor.
  Author(s): Hubble JP, Busenbark KL, Wilkinson S, Penn RD, Lyons K, Koller WC.
  Source: Neurology. 1996 April; 46(4): 1150-3.
  http://www.ncbi.nlm.nih.gov/entrez/query.fcgi?cmd=Retrieve&db=pubmed&dopt=Abstract&list_uids=8780109

- **Deep brain stimulation holidays in essential tremor.**
  Author(s): Garcia Ruiz P, Muniz de Igneson J, Lopez Ferro O, Martin C, Magarinos Ascone C.
  Source: Journal of Neurology. 2001 August; 248(8): 725-6.
  http://www.ncbi.nlm.nih.gov/entrez/query.fcgi?cmd=Retrieve&db=pubmed&dopt=A bstract&list_uids=11569910

- **Deep brain stimulation of the ventral intermediate nucleus of the thalamus for control of tremors in Parkinson's disease and essential tremor.**
  Author(s): Kumar K, Kelly M, Toth C.
  Source: Stereotactic and Functional Neurosurgery. 1999; 72(1): 47-61.
  http://www.ncbi.nlm.nih.gov/entrez/query.fcgi?cmd=Retrieve&db=pubmed&dopt=A bstract&list_uids=10640920

- **Deep brain stimulation of the VIM thalamic nucleus modifies several features of essential tremor.**
  Author(s): Vaillancourt DE, Sturman MM, Verhagen Metman L, Bakay RA, Corcos DM.
  Source: Neurology. 2003 October 14; 61(7): 919-25.
  http://www.ncbi.nlm.nih.gov/entrez/query.fcgi?cmd=Retrieve&db=pubmed&dopt=A bstract&list_uids=14557560

- **Diagnostic criteria for essential tremor and differential diagnosis.**
  Author(s): Elble RJ.
  Source: Neurology. 2000; 54(11 Suppl 4): S2-6.
  http://www.ncbi.nlm.nih.gov/entrez/query.fcgi?cmd=Retrieve&db=pubmed&dopt=A bstract&list_uids=10854344

- **Diagnostic criteria for essential tremor: a population perspective.**
  Author(s): Louis ED, Ford B, Lee H, Andrews H, Cameron G.
  Source: Archives of Neurology. 1998 June; 55(6): 823-8.
  http://www.ncbi.nlm.nih.gov/entrez/query.fcgi?cmd=Retrieve&db=pubmed&dopt=A bstract&list_uids=9626774

- **Difference of disability between electrophysiologic subgroups of essential tremor.**
  Author(s): Akbostanci MC, Ulkatan S, Yigit A, Aydin N, Mutluer N.
  Source: The Canadian Journal of Neurological Sciences. Le Journal Canadien Des Sciences Neurologiques. 2000 February; 27(1): 60-4.
  http://www.ncbi.nlm.nih.gov/entrez/query.fcgi?cmd=Retrieve&db=pubmed&dopt=A bstract&list_uids=10676590

- **Differences in the prevalence of essential tremor among elderly African Americans, whites, and Hispanics in northern Manhattan, NY.**
  Author(s): Louis ED, Marder K, Cote L, Pullman S, Ford B, Wilder D, Tang MX, Lantigua R, Gurland B, Mayeux R.
  Source: Archives of Neurology. 1995 December; 52(12): 1201-5.
  http://www.ncbi.nlm.nih.gov/entrez/query.fcgi?cmd=Retrieve&db=pubmed&dopt=A bstract&list_uids=7492295

- **Different clinical features of essential tremor: a 200-patient study.**
  Author(s): Martinelli P, Gabellini AS, Gulli MR, Lugaresi E.
  Source: Acta Neurologica Scandinavica. 1987 February; 75(2): 106-11.
  http://www.ncbi.nlm.nih.gov/entrez/query.fcgi?cmd=Retrieve&db=pubmed&dopt=Abstract&list_uids=3577675

- **Disability in essential tremor: effect of treatment.**
  Author(s): Koller W, Biary N, Cone S.
  Source: Neurology. 1986 July; 36(7): 1001-4.
  http://www.ncbi.nlm.nih.gov/entrez/query.fcgi?cmd=Retrieve&db=pubmed&dopt=Abstract&list_uids=2940473

- **Disappearance of essential tremor after small thalamic hemorrhage.**
  Author(s): Im JH, Kim JS, Lee MC.
  Source: Clinical Neurology and Neurosurgery. 1996 February; 98(1): 40-2.
  http://www.ncbi.nlm.nih.gov/entrez/query.fcgi?cmd=Retrieve&db=pubmed&dopt=Abstract&list_uids=8681478

- **Does a screening questionnaire for essential tremor agree with the physician's examination?**
  Author(s): Louis ED, Ford B, Lee H, Andrews H.
  Source: Neurology. 1998 May; 50(5): 1351-7.
  http://www.ncbi.nlm.nih.gov/entrez/query.fcgi?cmd=Retrieve&db=pubmed&dopt=Abstract&list_uids=9595986

- **Does essential tremor originate in the cerebral cortex?**
  Author(s): McAuley JH.
  Source: Lancet. 2001 February 17; 357(9255): 492-4.
  http://www.ncbi.nlm.nih.gov/entrez/query.fcgi?cmd=Retrieve&db=pubmed&dopt=Abstract&list_uids=11229663

- **Dose-response relationship of propranolol in the treatment of essential tremor.**
  Author(s): Koller WC.
  Source: Archives of Neurology. 1986 January; 43(1): 42-3.
  http://www.ncbi.nlm.nih.gov/entrez/query.fcgi?cmd=Retrieve&db=pubmed&dopt=Abstract&list_uids=3942513

- **Double-blind comparison of primidone and phenobarbital in essential tremor.**
  Author(s): Sasso E, Perucca E, Calzetti S.
  Source: Neurology. 1988 May; 38(5): 808-10.
  http://www.ncbi.nlm.nih.gov/entrez/query.fcgi?cmd=Retrieve&db=pubmed&dopt=Abstract&list_uids=3283599

- **Double-blind controlled study of methazolamide in the treatment of essential tremor.**
  Author(s): Busenbark K, Pahwa R, Hubble J, Hopfensperger K, Koller W, Pogrebra K.
  Source: Neurology. 1993 May; 43(5): 1045-7. Erratum In: Neurology 1993 October; 43(10): 1910.
  http://www.ncbi.nlm.nih.gov/entrez/query.fcgi?cmd=Retrieve&db=pubmed&dopt=Abstract&list_uids=8492925

- **Double-blind controlled trial of gabapentin in essential tremor.**
  Author(s): Pahwa R, Lyons K, Hubble JP, Busenbark K, Rienerth JD, Pahwa A, Koller WC.
  Source: Movement Disorders : Official Journal of the Movement Disorder Society. 1998 May; 13(3): 465-7.
  http://www.ncbi.nlm.nih.gov/entrez/query.fcgi?cmd=Retrieve&db=pubmed&dopt=Abstract&list_uids=9613738

- **Dual channel deep brain stimulation system (Kinetra) for Parkinson's disease and essential tremor: a prospective multicentre open label clinical study.**
  Author(s): Vesper J, Chabardes S, Fraix V, Sunde N, Ostergaard K; Kinetra Study Group.
  Source: Journal of Neurology, Neurosurgery, and Psychiatry. 2002 September; 73(3): 275-80.
  http://www.ncbi.nlm.nih.gov/entrez/query.fcgi?cmd=Retrieve&db=pubmed&dopt=Abstract&list_uids=12185158

- **Duration of effectiveness of primidone in essential tremor.**
  Author(s): Crystal HA.
  Source: Neurology. 1986 November; 36(11): 1543.
  http://www.ncbi.nlm.nih.gov/entrez/query.fcgi?cmd=Retrieve&db=pubmed&dopt=Abstract&list_uids=3762978

- **Dynamic synchronisation of central oscillators in essential tremor.**
  Author(s): Hellwig B, Schelter B, Guschlbauer B, Timmer J, Lucking CH.
  Source: Clinical Neurophysiology : Official Journal of the International Federation of Clinical Neurophysiology. 2003 August; 114(8): 1462-7.
  http://www.ncbi.nlm.nih.gov/entrez/query.fcgi?cmd=Retrieve&db=pubmed&dopt=Abstract&list_uids=12888029

- **Effect of ethanol on the central oscillator in essential tremor.**
  Author(s): Zeuner KE, Molloy FM, Shoge RO, Goldstein SR, Wesley R, Hallett M.
  Source: Movement Disorders : Official Journal of the Movement Disorder Society. 2003 November; 18(11): 1280-5.
  http://www.ncbi.nlm.nih.gov/entrez/query.fcgi?cmd=Retrieve&db=pubmed&dopt=Abstract&list_uids=14639668

- **Effective treatment for essential tremor.**
  Author(s): Young RR.
  Source: Annals of Neurology. 2002 March; 51(3): 407.
  http://www.ncbi.nlm.nih.gov/entrez/query.fcgi?cmd=Retrieve&db=pubmed&dopt=Abstract&list_uids=11891840

- **Electrophysiological approach to the study of essential tremor in children and adolescents.**
  Author(s): Fusco C, Valls-Sole J, Iturriaga C, Colomer J, Fernandez-Alvarez E.
  Source: Developmental Medicine and Child Neurology. 2003 September; 45(9): 624-7.
  http://www.ncbi.nlm.nih.gov/entrez/query.fcgi?cmd=Retrieve&db=pubmed&dopt=Abstract&list_uids=12948330

- **Elevation of blood beta-carboline alkaloids in essential tremor.**
  Author(s): Louis ED, Zheng W, Jurewicz EC, Watner D, Chen J, Factor-Litvak P, Parides M.
  Source: Neurology. 2002 December 24; 59(12): 1940-4.
  http://www.ncbi.nlm.nih.gov/entrez/query.fcgi?cmd=Retrieve&db=pubmed&dopt=Abstract&list_uids=12499487

- **Emergence of complex, involuntary movements after gamma knife radiosurgery for essential tremor.**
  Author(s): Siderowf A, Gollump SM, Stern MB, Baltuch GH, Riina HA.
  Source: Movement Disorders : Official Journal of the Movement Disorder Society. 2001 September; 16(5): 965-7.
  http://www.ncbi.nlm.nih.gov/entrez/query.fcgi?cmd=Retrieve&db=pubmed&dopt=Abstract&list_uids=11746633

- **Essential tremor and cerebellar dysfunction: abnormal ballistic movements.**
  Author(s): Koster B, Deuschl G, Lauk M, Timmer J, Guschlbauer B, Lucking CH.
  Source: Journal of Neurology, Neurosurgery, and Psychiatry. 2002 October; 73(4): 400-5.
  http://www.ncbi.nlm.nih.gov/entrez/query.fcgi?cmd=Retrieve&db=pubmed&dopt=Abstract&list_uids=12235308

- **Essential tremor and parkinsonism.**
  Author(s): Rajput A, Rajput M.
  Source: Adv Neurol. 2003; 91: 397-9. Review. No Abstract Available.
  http://www.ncbi.nlm.nih.gov/entrez/query.fcgi?cmd=Retrieve&db=pubmed&dopt=Abstract&list_uids=12442698

- **Essential tremor course and disability: A clinicopathologic study of 20 cases.**
  Author(s): Rajput A, Robinson CA, Rajput AH.
  Source: Neurology. 2004 March 23; 62(6): 932-6.
  http://www.ncbi.nlm.nih.gov/entrez/query.fcgi?cmd=Retrieve&db=pubmed&dopt=Abstract&list_uids=15037695

- **Essential tremor in childhood: a series of nineteen cases.**
  Author(s): Louis ED, Dure LS 4th, Pullman S.
  Source: Movement Disorders : Official Journal of the Movement Disorder Society. 2001 September; 16(5): 921-3.
  http://www.ncbi.nlm.nih.gov/entrez/query.fcgi?cmd=Retrieve&db=pubmed&dopt=Abstract&list_uids=11746623

- **Essential tremor in twins: an assessment of genetic vs environmental determinants of etiology.**
  Author(s): Tanner CM, Goldman SM, Lyons KE, Aston DA, Tetrud JW, Welsh MD, Langston JW, Koller WC.
  Source: Neurology. 2001 October 23; 57(8): 1389-91.
  http://www.ncbi.nlm.nih.gov/entrez/query.fcgi?cmd=Retrieve&db=pubmed&dopt=Abstract&list_uids=11673577

- **Essential tremor is a monosymptomatic disorder.**
  Author(s): Elble RJ.
  Source: Movement Disorders : Official Journal of the Movement Disorder Society. 2002 July; 17(4): 633-7. Review.
  http://www.ncbi.nlm.nih.gov/entrez/query.fcgi?cmd=Retrieve&db=pubmed&dopt=Abstract&list_uids=12210850

- **Essential tremor is not associated with alpha-synuclein gene haplotypes.**
  Author(s): Pigullo S, Di Maria E, Marchese R, Bellone E, Gulli R, Scaglione C, Battaglia S, Barone P, Martinelli P, Abbruzzese G, Ajmar F, Mandich P.
  Source: Movement Disorders : Official Journal of the Movement Disorder Society. 2003 July; 18(7): 823-6.
  http://www.ncbi.nlm.nih.gov/entrez/query.fcgi?cmd=Retrieve&db=pubmed&dopt=Abstract&list_uids=12815663

- **Essential tremor.**
  Author(s): Sampaio C, Ferreira J.
  Source: Clin Evid. 2002 June; (7): 1169-78. Review. No Abstract Available.
  http://www.ncbi.nlm.nih.gov/entrez/query.fcgi?cmd=Retrieve&db=pubmed&dopt=Abstract&list_uids=12230735

- **Essential tremor.**
  Author(s): van den Noort S.
  Source: The New England Journal of Medicine. 2002 February 28; 346(9): 709-10.
  http://www.ncbi.nlm.nih.gov/entrez/query.fcgi?cmd=Retrieve&db=pubmed&dopt=Abstract&list_uids=11870253

- **Essential tremor: a heterogenous disorder.**
  Author(s): Jankovic J.
  Source: Movement Disorders : Official Journal of the Movement Disorder Society. 2002 July; 17(4): 638-44. Review.
  http://www.ncbi.nlm.nih.gov/entrez/query.fcgi?cmd=Retrieve&db=pubmed&dopt=Abstract&list_uids=12210851

- **Essential tremor: diagnosis and treatment.**
  Author(s): Chen JJ, Swope DM.
  Source: Pharmacotherapy. 2003 September; 23(9): 1105-22. Review.
  http://www.ncbi.nlm.nih.gov/entrez/query.fcgi?cmd=Retrieve&db=pubmed&dopt=Abstract&list_uids=14524643

- **Essential tremor: differential diagnosis and current therapy.**
  Author(s): Pahwa R, Lyons KE.
  Source: The American Journal of Medicine. 2003 August 1; 115(2): 134-42. Review.
  http://www.ncbi.nlm.nih.gov/entrez/query.fcgi?cmd=Retrieve&db=pubmed&dopt=Abstract&list_uids=12893400

- **Etiology of essential tremor: should we be searching for environmental causes?**
  Author(s): Louis ED.
  Source: Movement Disorders : Official Journal of the Movement Disorder Society. 2001 September; 16(5): 822-9. Review.
  http://www.ncbi.nlm.nih.gov/entrez/query.fcgi?cmd=Retrieve&db=pubmed&dopt=Abstract&list_uids=11746611

- **Evaluation of essential tremor with multi-voxel magnetic resonance spectroscopy.**
  Author(s): Pagan FL, Butman JA, Dambrosia JM, Hallett M.
  Source: Neurology. 2003 April 22; 60(8): 1344-7.
  http://www.ncbi.nlm.nih.gov/entrez/query.fcgi?cmd=Retrieve&db=pubmed&dopt=Abstract&list_uids=12707440

- **Eye movement abnormalities in essential tremor may indicate cerebellar dysfunction.**
  Author(s): Helmchen C, Hagenow A, Miesner J, Sprenger A, Rambold H, Wenzelburger R, Heide W, Deuschl G.
  Source: Brain; a Journal of Neurology. 2003 June; 126(Pt 6): 1319-32.
  http://www.ncbi.nlm.nih.gov/entrez/query.fcgi?cmd=Retrieve&db=pubmed&dopt=Abstract&list_uids=12764054

- **Factors associated with increased risk of head tremor in essential tremor: a community-based study in northern Manhattan.**
  Author(s): Louis ED, Ford B, Frucht S.
  Source: Movement Disorders : Official Journal of the Movement Disorder Society. 2003 April; 18(4): 432-6.
  http://www.ncbi.nlm.nih.gov/entrez/query.fcgi?cmd=Retrieve&db=pubmed&dopt=Abstract&list_uids=12671952

- **Factors influencing the amplitude and frequency of essential tremor.**
  Author(s): Elble RJ, Higgins C, Leffler K, Hughes L.
  Source: Movement Disorders : Official Journal of the Movement Disorder Society. 1994 November; 9(6): 589-96. Erratum In: Mov Disord 1995 May; 10(3): 411.
  http://www.ncbi.nlm.nih.gov/entrez/query.fcgi?cmd=Retrieve&db=pubmed&dopt=Abstract&list_uids=7845397

- **Familial essential tremor and idiopathic torsion dystonia are different genetic entities.**
  Author(s): Durr A, Stevanin G, Jedynak CP, Penet C, Agid Y, Brice A.
  Source: Neurology. 1993 November; 43(11): 2212-4.
  http://www.ncbi.nlm.nih.gov/entrez/query.fcgi?cmd=Retrieve&db=pubmed&dopt=Abstract&list_uids=8232931

- **Familial essential tremor in 4 kindreds. Prospects for genetic mapping.**
  Author(s): Jankovic J, Beach J, Pandolfo M, Patel PI.
  Source: Archives of Neurology. 1997 March; 54(3): 289-94.
  http://www.ncbi.nlm.nih.gov/entrez/query.fcgi?cmd=Retrieve&db=pubmed&dopt=Abstract&list_uids=9074398

- **Familial essential tremor is not associated with SCA-12 mutation in southern Italy.**
  Author(s): Nicoletti G, Annesi G, Carrideo S, Tomaino C, Di Costanzo A, Zappia M, Quattrone A.
  Source: Movement Disorders : Official Journal of the Movement Disorder Society. 2002 July; 17(4): 837-8.
  http://www.ncbi.nlm.nih.gov/entrez/query.fcgi?cmd=Retrieve&db=pubmed&dopt=Abstract&list_uids=12210890

- **Familial migraine with vertigo and essential tremor.**
  Author(s): Baloh RW, Foster CA, Yue Q, Nelson SF.
  Source: Neurology. 1996 February; 46(2): 458-60.
  http://www.ncbi.nlm.nih.gov/entrez/query.fcgi?cmd=Retrieve&db=pubmed&dopt=Abstract&list_uids=8614512

- **Familial paroxysmal tremor: an essential tremor variant.**
  Author(s): Bain PG, Findley LJ.
  Source: Journal of Neurology, Neurosurgery, and Psychiatry. 1994 August; 57(8): 1019. Review.
  http://www.ncbi.nlm.nih.gov/entrez/query.fcgi?cmd=Retrieve&db=pubmed&dopt=Abstract&list_uids=8057106

- **Family history information on essential tremor: potential biases related to the source of the cases.**
  Author(s): Louis ED, Barnes LF, Ford B, Ottman R.
  Source: Movement Disorders : Official Journal of the Movement Disorder Society. 2001 March; 16(2): 320-4.
  http://www.ncbi.nlm.nih.gov/entrez/query.fcgi?cmd=Retrieve&db=pubmed&dopt=Abstract&list_uids=11295788

- **Flunarizine and essential tremor.**
  Author(s): Jimenez-Jimenez FJ, Garcia-Ruiz PJ.
  Source: Neurology. 1993 January; 43(1): 239.
  http://www.ncbi.nlm.nih.gov/entrez/query.fcgi?cmd=Retrieve&db=pubmed&dopt=Abstract&list_uids=8481198

- **Flunarizine in essential tremor.**
  Author(s): Curran T, Lang AE.
  Source: Clinical Neuropharmacology. 1993 October; 16(5): 460-3.
  http://www.ncbi.nlm.nih.gov/entrez/query.fcgi?cmd=Retrieve&db=pubmed&dopt=Abstract&list_uids=8221708

- **Frequency/amplitude characteristics of postural tremor of the hands in a population of patients with bilateral essential tremor: implications for the classification and mechanism of essential tremor.**
  Author(s): Calzetti S, Baratti M, Gresty M, Findley L.
  Source: Journal of Neurology, Neurosurgery, and Psychiatry. 1987 May; 50(5): 561-7.
  http://www.ncbi.nlm.nih.gov/entrez/query.fcgi?cmd=Retrieve&db=pubmed&dopt=Abstract&list_uids=3585381

- **Frontal lobe dysfunction in essential tremor: a preliminary study.**
  Author(s): Gasparini M, Bonifati V, Fabrizio E, Fabbrini G, Brusa L, Lenzi GL, Meco G.
  Source: Journal of Neurology. 2001 May; 248(5): 399-402.
  http://www.ncbi.nlm.nih.gov/entrez/query.fcgi?cmd=Retrieve&db=pubmed&dopt=Abstract&list_uids=11437162

- **Functional outcomes after gamma knife thalamotomy for essential tremor and MS-related tremor.**
  Author(s): Niranjan A, Kondziolka D, Baser S, Heyman R, Lunsford LD.
  Source: Neurology. 2000 August 8; 55(3): 443-6.
  http://www.ncbi.nlm.nih.gov/entrez/query.fcgi?cmd=Retrieve&db=pubmed&dopt=Abstract&list_uids=10932286

- **Gabapentin for essential tremor: a multiple-dose, double-blind, placebo-controlled trial.**
  Author(s): Ondo W, Hunter C, Vuong KD, Schwartz K, Jankovic J.
  Source: Movement Disorders : Official Journal of the Movement Disorder Society. 2000 July; 15(4): 678-82.
  http://www.ncbi.nlm.nih.gov/entrez/query.fcgi?cmd=Retrieve&db=pubmed&dopt=Abstract&list_uids=10928578

- **Gait abnormality in essential tremor.**
  Author(s): Singer C, Sanchez-Ramos J, Weiner WJ.
  Source: Movement Disorders : Official Journal of the Movement Disorder Society. 1994 March; 9(2): 193-6.
  http://www.ncbi.nlm.nih.gov/entrez/query.fcgi?cmd=Retrieve&db=pubmed&dopt=Abstract&list_uids=8196682

- **Genetic heterogeneity in autosomal dominant essential tremor.**
  Author(s): Kovach MJ, Ruiz J, Kimonis K, Mueed S, Sinha S, Higgins C, Elble S, Elble R, Kimonis VE.
  Source: Genetics in Medicine : Official Journal of the American College of Medical Genetics. 2001 May-June; 3(3): 197-9.
  http://www.ncbi.nlm.nih.gov/entrez/query.fcgi?cmd=Retrieve&db=pubmed&dopt=Abstract&list_uids=11388761

- **Glucose metabolism in the brain of patients with essential tremor.**
  Author(s): Hallett M, Dubinsky RM.
  Source: Journal of the Neurological Sciences. 1993 January; 114(1): 45-8.
  http://www.ncbi.nlm.nih.gov/entrez/query.fcgi?cmd=Retrieve&db=pubmed&dopt=Abstract&list_uids=8433096

- **Grasping essential tremor.**
  Author(s): Plotkin G.
  Source: Health News. 1999 October 1; 5(12): 1-2. No Abstract Available.
  http://www.ncbi.nlm.nih.gov/entrez/query.fcgi?cmd=Retrieve&db=pubmed&dopt=Abstract&list_uids=10536527

- **Handedness and essential tremor.**
  Author(s): Biary N, Koller W.
  Source: Archives of Neurology. 1985 November; 42(11): 1082-3.
  http://www.ncbi.nlm.nih.gov/entrez/query.fcgi?cmd=Retrieve&db=pubmed&dopt=Abstract&list_uids=4051838

- **Haplotype analysis of the ETM2 locus in familial essential tremor.**
  Author(s): Higgins JJ, Jankovic J, Lombardi RQ, Pucilowska J, Tan EK, Ashizawa T, Ruszczyk MU.
  Source: Neurogenetics. 2003 August; 4(4): 185-9. Epub 2003 May 22.
  http://www.ncbi.nlm.nih.gov/entrez/query.fcgi?cmd=Retrieve&db=pubmed&dopt=Abstract&list_uids=12761658

- **Hereditary essential tremor and restless legs syndrome.**
  Author(s): Larner AJ, Allen CM.
  Source: Postgraduate Medical Journal. 1997 April; 73(858): 254.
  http://www.ncbi.nlm.nih.gov/entrez/query.fcgi?cmd=Retrieve&db=pubmed&dopt=Abstract&list_uids=9156136

- **Hereditary essential tremor in Buenos Aires (Argentina).**
  Author(s): Herskovits E, Figueroa E, Mangone C.
  Source: Arquivos De Neuro-Psiquiatria. 1988 September; 46(3): 238-47.
  http://www.ncbi.nlm.nih.gov/entrez/query.fcgi?cmd=Retrieve&db=pubmed&dopt=Abstract&list_uids=3223829

- **High alcoholism rate in patients with essential tremor.**
  Author(s): Schroeder D, Nasrallah HA.
  Source: The American Journal of Psychiatry. 1982 November; 139(11): 1471-3.
  http://www.ncbi.nlm.nih.gov/entrez/query.fcgi?cmd=Retrieve&db=pubmed&dopt=Abstract&list_uids=7137398

- **Homolateral disappearance of essential tremor after cerebellar stroke.**
  Author(s): Dupuis MJ, Delwaide PJ, Boucquey D, Gonsette RE.
  Source: Movement Disorders : Official Journal of the Movement Disorder Society. 1989; 4(2): 183-7.
  http://www.ncbi.nlm.nih.gov/entrez/query.fcgi?cmd=Retrieve&db=pubmed&dopt=Abstract&list_uids=2733709

- **How common is the most common adult movement disorder? estimates of the prevalence of essential tremor throughout the world.**
  Author(s): Louis ED, Ottman R, Hauser WA.
  Source: Movement Disorders : Official Journal of the Movement Disorder Society. 1998 January; 13(1): 5-10. Review.
  http://www.ncbi.nlm.nih.gov/entrez/query.fcgi?cmd=Retrieve&db=pubmed&dopt=Abstract&list_uids=9452318

- **How familial is familial tremor? The genetic epidemiology of essential tremor.**
  Author(s): Louis ED, Ottman R.
  Source: Neurology. 1996 May; 46(5): 1200-5. Review.
  http://www.ncbi.nlm.nih.gov/entrez/query.fcgi?cmd=Retrieve&db=pubmed&dopt=A
  bstract&list_uids=8628453

- **H-reflex recovery curves differentiate essential tremor, Parkinson's disease, and the combination of essential tremor and Parkinson's disease.**
  Author(s): Sabbahi M, Etnyre B, Al-Jawayed I, Jankovic J.
  Source: Journal of Clinical Neurophysiology : Official Publication of the American Electroencephalographic Society. 2002 June; 19(3): 245-51.
  http://www.ncbi.nlm.nih.gov/entrez/query.fcgi?cmd=Retrieve&db=pubmed&dopt=A
  bstract&list_uids=12226570

- **Hypotonia accompanying the neurosurgical relief of essential tremor.**
  Author(s): Blacker HM, Bertrand C, Martinez N, Hardy J, Molina-Negro P.
  Source: The Journal of Nervous and Mental Disease. 1968 July; 147(1): 49-55.
  http://www.ncbi.nlm.nih.gov/entrez/query.fcgi?cmd=Retrieve&db=pubmed&dopt=A
  bstract&list_uids=4875661

- **Impact of thalamic deep brain stimulation on disability and health-related quality of life in patients with essential tremor.**
  Author(s): Hariz GM, Lindberg M, Bergenheim AT.
  Source: Journal of Neurology, Neurosurgery, and Psychiatry. 2002 January; 72(1): 47-52.
  http://www.ncbi.nlm.nih.gov/entrez/query.fcgi?cmd=Retrieve&db=pubmed&dopt=A
  bstract&list_uids=11784825

- **Improvement in essential tremor after pure sensory stroke due to thalamic infarction.**
  Author(s): Barbaud A, Hadjout K, Blard JM, Pages M.
  Source: European Neurology. 2001; 46(1): 57-9.
  http://www.ncbi.nlm.nih.gov/entrez/query.fcgi?cmd=Retrieve&db=pubmed&dopt=A
  bstract&list_uids=11455190

- **Ineffective treatment of essential tremor with an alcohol, methylpentynol.**
  Author(s): Teravainen H, Huttunen J, Lewitt P.
  Source: Journal of Neurology, Neurosurgery, and Psychiatry. 1986 February; 49(2): 198-9.
  http://www.ncbi.nlm.nih.gov/entrez/query.fcgi?cmd=Retrieve&db=pubmed&dopt=A
  bstract&list_uids=3512778

- **Ineffectiveness of phenoxybenzamine in essential tremor.**
  Author(s): Koller WC.
  Source: Journal of Neurology, Neurosurgery, and Psychiatry. 1986 February; 49(2): 222.
  http://www.ncbi.nlm.nih.gov/entrez/query.fcgi?cmd=Retrieve&db=pubmed&dopt=A
  bstract&list_uids=3950649

- **Inefficacy of tryptophan-pyridoxine in essential tremor.**
  Author(s): Mozzis CE, Prange AJ Jr, Hall CD, Weiss EA.
  Source: Lancet. 1971 July 17; 2(7716): 165-6.
  http://www.ncbi.nlm.nih.gov/entrez/query.fcgi?cmd=Retrieve&db=pubmed&dopt=A bstract&list_uids=4104493

- **Introduction. Essential tremor.**
  Author(s): Deuschl G, Koller WC.
  Source: Neurology. 2000; 54(11 Suppl 4): S1.
  http://www.ncbi.nlm.nih.gov/entrez/query.fcgi?cmd=Retrieve&db=pubmed&dopt=A bstract&list_uids=10854343

- **Ipsilateral thalamic stimulation after thalamotomy for essential tremor. A case report.**
  Author(s): Racette BA, Rich KM, Randle J, Mink JW.
  Source: Stereotactic and Functional Neurosurgery. 2000; 75(4): 155-9.
  http://www.ncbi.nlm.nih.gov/entrez/query.fcgi?cmd=Retrieve&db=pubmed&dopt=A bstract&list_uids=11910208

- **Is essential tremor benign?**
  Author(s): Busenbark KL, Nash J, Nash S, Hubble JP, Koller WC.
  Source: Neurology. 1991 December; 41(12): 1982-3.
  http://www.ncbi.nlm.nih.gov/entrez/query.fcgi?cmd=Retrieve&db=pubmed&dopt=A bstract&list_uids=1745359

- **Is essential tremor predominantly a kinetic or a postural tremor? A clinical and electrophysiological study.**
  Author(s): Brennan KC, Jurewicz EC, Ford B, Pullman SL, Louis ED.
  Source: Movement Disorders : Official Journal of the Movement Disorder Society. 2002 March; 17(2): 313-6.
  http://www.ncbi.nlm.nih.gov/entrez/query.fcgi?cmd=Retrieve&db=pubmed&dopt=A bstract&list_uids=11921117

- **Is essential tremor symmetric? Observational data from a community-based study of essential tremor.**
  Author(s): Louis ED, Wendt KJ, Pullman SL, Ford B.
  Source: Archives of Neurology. 1998 December; 55(12): 1553-9.
  http://www.ncbi.nlm.nih.gov/entrez/query.fcgi?cmd=Retrieve&db=pubmed&dopt=A bstract&list_uids=9865800

- **Is there a relationship between Parkinson's disease and essential tremor?**
  Author(s): Pahwa R, Koller WC.
  Source: Clinical Neuropharmacology. 1993 February; 16(1): 30-5. Review.
  http://www.ncbi.nlm.nih.gov/entrez/query.fcgi?cmd=Retrieve&db=pubmed&dopt=A bstract&list_uids=8422655

- **Issues relating to functional disability in essential tremor.**
  Author(s): Louis ED.
  Source: The Canadian Journal of Neurological Sciences. Le Journal Canadien Des Sciences Neurologiques. 2000 November; 27(4): 354.
  http://www.ncbi.nlm.nih.gov/entrez/query.fcgi?cmd=Retrieve&db=pubmed&dopt=Abstract&list_uids=11097531

- **Kinetic predominant essential tremor: successful treatment with clonazepam.**
  Author(s): Biary N, Koller W.
  Source: Neurology. 1987 March; 37(3): 471-4.
  http://www.ncbi.nlm.nih.gov/entrez/query.fcgi?cmd=Retrieve&db=pubmed&dopt=Abstract&list_uids=3822141

- **Klinefelter's syndrome and essential tremor.**
  Author(s): Baughman FA Jr.
  Source: Lancet. 1969 September 6; 2(7619): 545.
  http://www.ncbi.nlm.nih.gov/entrez/query.fcgi?cmd=Retrieve&db=pubmed&dopt=Abstract&list_uids=4184860

- **Lack of association between essential tremor and Parkinson's disease.**
  Author(s): Cleeves L, Findley LJ, Koller W.
  Source: Annals of Neurology. 1988 July; 24(1): 23-6.
  http://www.ncbi.nlm.nih.gov/entrez/query.fcgi?cmd=Retrieve&db=pubmed&dopt=Abstract&list_uids=3415197

- **Letter: Shuddering attacks in children: essential tremor and monosodium glutamate.**
  Author(s): Andermann F, Vanasse M, Wolfe LS.
  Source: The New England Journal of Medicine. 1976 July 15; 295(3): 174.
  http://www.ncbi.nlm.nih.gov/entrez/query.fcgi?cmd=Retrieve&db=pubmed&dopt=Abstract&list_uids=1272343

- **Limb positioning and magnitude of essential tremor and other pathological tremors.**
  Author(s): Sanes JN, Hallett M.
  Source: Movement Disorders : Official Journal of the Movement Disorder Society. 1990; 5(4): 304-9.
  http://www.ncbi.nlm.nih.gov/entrez/query.fcgi?cmd=Retrieve&db=pubmed&dopt=Abstract&list_uids=2259353

- **Linkage analysis with chromosome 9 markers in hereditary essential tremor.**
  Author(s): Conway D, Bain PG, Warner TT, Davis MB, Findley LJ, Thompson PD, Marsden CD, Harding AE.
  Source: Movement Disorders : Official Journal of the Movement Disorder Society. 1993 July; 8(3): 374-6.
  http://www.ncbi.nlm.nih.gov/entrez/query.fcgi?cmd=Retrieve&db=pubmed&dopt=Abstract&list_uids=8341306

- **Localization of thalamic cells with tremor-frequency activity in Parkinson's disease and essential tremor.**
  Author(s): Kobayashi K, Katayama Y, Kasai M, Oshima H, Fukaya C, Yamamoto T.
  Source: Acta Neurochir Suppl. 2003; 87: 137-9.
  http://www.ncbi.nlm.nih.gov/entrez/query.fcgi?cmd=Retrieve&db=pubmed&dopt=Abstract&list_uids=14518541

- **Long-acting propranolol in essential tremor.**
  Author(s): Koller WC.
  Source: Neurology. 1985 January; 35(1): 108-10.
  http://www.ncbi.nlm.nih.gov/entrez/query.fcgi?cmd=Retrieve&db=pubmed&dopt=Abstract&list_uids=3965982

- **Longitudinal study of essential tremor.**
  Author(s): Elble RJ, Higgins C, Hughes L.
  Source: Neurology. 1992 February; 42(2): 441-3.
  http://www.ncbi.nlm.nih.gov/entrez/query.fcgi?cmd=Retrieve&db=pubmed&dopt=Abstract&list_uids=1736181

- **Long-term deep brain stimulation in a patient with essential tremor: clinical response and postmortem correlation with stimulator termination sites in ventral thalamus. Case report.**
  Author(s): Boockvar JA, Telfeian A, Baltuch GH, Skolnick B, Simuni T, Stern M, Schmidt ML, Trojanowski JQ.
  Source: Journal of Neurosurgery. 2000 July; 93(1): 140-4.
  http://www.ncbi.nlm.nih.gov/entrez/query.fcgi?cmd=Retrieve&db=pubmed&dopt=Abstract&list_uids=10883919

- **Long-term results of stereotaxy in the treatment of essential tremor.**
  Author(s): Mohadjer M, Goerke H, Milios E, Etou A, Mundinger F.
  Source: Stereotactic and Functional Neurosurgery. 1990; 54-55: 125-9.
  http://www.ncbi.nlm.nih.gov/entrez/query.fcgi?cmd=Retrieve&db=pubmed&dopt=Abstract&list_uids=2080326

- **Long-term safety and efficacy of unilateral deep brain stimulation of the thalamus in essential tremor.**
  Author(s): Koller WC, Lyons KE, Wilkinson SB, Troster AI, Pahwa R.
  Source: Movement Disorders : Official Journal of the Movement Disorder Society. 2001 May; 16(3): 464-8.
  http://www.ncbi.nlm.nih.gov/entrez/query.fcgi?cmd=Retrieve&db=pubmed&dopt=Abstract&list_uids=11391740

- **Long-term therapy of essential tremor with flunarizine.**
  Author(s): Biary N, al Deeb SM, Bahou Y.
  Source: European Neurology. 1995; 35(4): 217-9.
  http://www.ncbi.nlm.nih.gov/entrez/query.fcgi?cmd=Retrieve&db=pubmed&dopt=Abstract&list_uids=7671982

- **Long-term therapy of essential tremor with propranolol.**
  Author(s): Murray TJ.
  Source: Can Med Assoc J. 1976 November 6; 115(9): 892-4.
  http://www.ncbi.nlm.nih.gov/entrez/query.fcgi?cmd=Retrieve&db=pubmed&dopt=A
  bstract&list_uids=791468

- **Long-term tremor recordings in parkinsonian and essential tremor.**
  Author(s): Spieker S, Boose A, Jentgens C, Dichgans J.
  Source: Journal of Neural Transmission. Supplementum. 1995; 46: 339-49.
  http://www.ncbi.nlm.nih.gov/entrez/query.fcgi?cmd=Retrieve&db=pubmed&dopt=A
  bstract&list_uids=8821070

- **Loss of reflex inhibition following muscle tendon stimulation in essential tremor.**
  Author(s): Burne JA, Blanche T, Morris JG.
  Source: Muscle & Nerve. 2002 January; 25(1): 58-64.
  http://www.ncbi.nlm.nih.gov/entrez/query.fcgi?cmd=Retrieve&db=pubmed&dopt=A
  bstract&list_uids=11754186

- **Low doses of topiramate are effective in essential tremor: a report of three cases.**
  Author(s): Gatto EM, Roca MC, Raina G, Micheli F.
  Source: Clinical Neuropharmacology. 2003 November-December; 26(6): 294-6.
  http://www.ncbi.nlm.nih.gov/entrez/query.fcgi?cmd=Retrieve&db=pubmed&dopt=A
  bstract&list_uids=14646607

- **Mapping of a familial essential tremor gene, FET1, to chromosome 3q13.**
  Author(s): Gulcher JR, Jonsson P, Kong A, Kristjansson K, Frigge ML, Karason A,
  Einarsdottir IE, Stefansson H, Einarsdottir AS, Sigurthoardottir S, Baldursson S,
  Bjornsdottir S, Hrafnkelsdottir SM, Jakobsson F, Benedickz J, Stefansson K.
  Source: Nature Genetics. 1997 September; 17(1): 84-7.
  http://www.ncbi.nlm.nih.gov/entrez/query.fcgi?cmd=Retrieve&db=pubmed&dopt=A
  bstract&list_uids=9288103

- **Mechanisms for essential tremor.**
  Author(s): Britton TC, Gresty MA.
  Source: Lancet. 1992 September 5; 340(8819): 610.
  http://www.ncbi.nlm.nih.gov/entrez/query.fcgi?cmd=Retrieve&db=pubmed&dopt=A
  bstract&list_uids=1355182

- **Medical treatment of essential tremor and Parkinson's disease.**
  Author(s): Uitti RJ.
  Source: Geriatrics. 1998 May; 53(5): 46-8, 53-7. Review.
  http://www.ncbi.nlm.nih.gov/entrez/query.fcgi?cmd=Retrieve&db=pubmed&dopt=A
  bstract&list_uids=9597979

- **Metabolic abnormality in the cerebellum in patients with essential tremor: a proton
  magnetic resonance spectroscopic imaging study.**
  Author(s): Louis ED, Shungu DC, Chan S, Mao X, Jurewicz EC, Watner D.
  Source: Neuroscience Letters. 2002 November 15; 333(1): 17-20.
  http://www.ncbi.nlm.nih.gov/entrez/query.fcgi?cmd=Retrieve&db=pubmed&dopt=A
  bstract&list_uids=12401550

- **Metoprolol and alpha-hydroxymetoprolol concentrations and reduction in essential tremor.**
  Author(s): Gengo FM, Ulatowski JA, McHugh WB.
  Source: Clinical Pharmacology and Therapeutics. 1984 September; 36(3): 320-5.
  http://www.ncbi.nlm.nih.gov/entrez/query.fcgi?cmd=Retrieve&db=pubmed&dopt=Abstract&list_uids=6467791

- **Metoprolol and propranolol in essential tremor: a double-blind, controlled study.**
  Author(s): Calzetti S, Findley LJ, Gresty MA, Perucca E, Richens A.
  Source: Journal of Neurology, Neurosurgery, and Psychiatry. 1981 September; 44(9): 814-9.
  http://www.ncbi.nlm.nih.gov/entrez/query.fcgi?cmd=Retrieve&db=pubmed&dopt=Abstract&list_uids=7031187

- **Metoprolol compared with propranolol in the treatment of essential tremor.**
  Author(s): Koller WC, Biary N.
  Source: Archives of Neurology. 1984 February; 41(2): 171-2.
  http://www.ncbi.nlm.nih.gov/entrez/query.fcgi?cmd=Retrieve&db=pubmed&dopt=Abstract&list_uids=6691818

- **Metoprolol in essential tremor.**
  Author(s): Calzetti S, Findley LJ, Perucca E, Richens A.
  Source: Lancet. 1981 November 28; 2(8257): 1227.
  http://www.ncbi.nlm.nih.gov/entrez/query.fcgi?cmd=Retrieve&db=pubmed&dopt=Abstract&list_uids=6118649

- **Metoprolol in essential tremor.**
  Author(s): Newman RP, Jacobs L.
  Source: Archives of Neurology. 1980 September; 37(9): 596-7.
  http://www.ncbi.nlm.nih.gov/entrez/query.fcgi?cmd=Retrieve&db=pubmed&dopt=Abstract&list_uids=7417066

- **Mild tremor in relatives of patients with essential tremor: what does this tell us about the penetrance of the disease?**
  Author(s): Louis ED, Ford B, Frucht S, Ottman R.
  Source: Archives of Neurology. 2001 October; 58(10): 1584-9.
  http://www.ncbi.nlm.nih.gov/entrez/query.fcgi?cmd=Retrieve&db=pubmed&dopt=Abstract&list_uids=11594916

- **Mirtazapine in essential tremor: a double-blind, placebo-controlled pilot study.**
  Author(s): Pahwa R, Lyons KE.
  Source: Movement Disorders : Official Journal of the Movement Disorder Society. 2003 May; 18(5): 584-7.
  http://www.ncbi.nlm.nih.gov/entrez/query.fcgi?cmd=Retrieve&db=pubmed&dopt=Abstract&list_uids=12722174

- **Mirtazapine treats resting tremor, essential tremor, and levodopa-induced dyskinesias.**
  Author(s): Pact V, Giduz T.
  Source: Neurology. 1999 September 22; 53(5): 1154.
  http://www.ncbi.nlm.nih.gov/entrez/query.fcgi?cmd=Retrieve&db=pubmed&dopt=Abstract&list_uids=10496290

- **Modulation of postural tremors at the wrist by supramaximal electrical median nerve shocks in essential tremor, Parkinson's disease and normal subjects mimicking tremor.**
  Author(s): Britton TC, Thompson PD, Day BL, Rothwell JC, Findley LJ, Marsden CD.
  Source: Journal of Neurology, Neurosurgery, and Psychiatry. 1993 October; 56(10): 1085-9.
  http://www.ncbi.nlm.nih.gov/entrez/query.fcgi?cmd=Retrieve&db=pubmed&dopt=Abstract&list_uids=8410007

- **Modulation of postural wrist tremors by magnetic stimulation of the motor cortex in patients with Parkinson's disease or essential tremor and in normal subjects mimicking tremor.**
  Author(s): Britton TC, Thompson PD, Day BL, Rothwell JC, Findley LJ, Marsden CD.
  Source: Annals of Neurology. 1993 May; 33(5): 473-9.
  http://www.ncbi.nlm.nih.gov/entrez/query.fcgi?cmd=Retrieve&db=pubmed&dopt=Abstract&list_uids=8498824

- **Motor initiation and execution in essential tremor and Parkinson's disease.**
  Author(s): Montgomery EB Jr, Baker KB, Lyons K, Koller WC.
  Source: Movement Disorders : Official Journal of the Movement Disorder Society. 2000 May; 15(3): 511-5.
  http://www.ncbi.nlm.nih.gov/entrez/query.fcgi?cmd=Retrieve&db=pubmed&dopt=Abstract&list_uids=10830417

- **Multicentre European study of thalamic stimulation in essential tremor.**
  Author(s): Dick JP.
  Source: Journal of Neurology, Neurosurgery, and Psychiatry. 2003 October; 74(10): 1362-3.
  http://www.ncbi.nlm.nih.gov/entrez/query.fcgi?cmd=Retrieve&db=pubmed&dopt=Abstract&list_uids=14570826

- **Multicentre European study of thalamic stimulation in essential tremor: a six year follow up.**
  Author(s): Sydow O, Thobois S, Alesch F, Speelman JD.
  Source: Journal of Neurology, Neurosurgery, and Psychiatry. 2003 October; 74(10): 1387-91.
  http://www.ncbi.nlm.nih.gov/entrez/query.fcgi?cmd=Retrieve&db=pubmed&dopt=Abstract&list_uids=14570831

- **Multicentre European study of thalamic stimulation in parkinsonian and essential tremor.**
  Author(s): Limousin P, Speelman JD, Gielen F, Janssens M.
  Source: Journal of Neurology, Neurosurgery, and Psychiatry. 1999 March; 66(3): 289-96.
  http://www.ncbi.nlm.nih.gov/entrez/query.fcgi?cmd=Retrieve&db=pubmed&dopt=Abstract&list_uids=10084526

- **Multiple oscillators are causing parkinsonian and essential tremor.**
  Author(s): Raethjen J, Lindemann M, Schmaljohann H, Wenzelburger R, Pfister G, Deuschl G.
  Source: Movement Disorders : Official Journal of the Movement Disorder Society. 2000 January; 15(1): 84-94.
  http://www.ncbi.nlm.nih.gov/entrez/query.fcgi?cmd=Retrieve&db=pubmed&dopt=Abstract&list_uids=10634246

- **Nadolol in essential tremor.**
  Author(s): Koller WC.
  Source: Neurology. 1983 August; 33(8): 1076-7.
  http://www.ncbi.nlm.nih.gov/entrez/query.fcgi?cmd=Retrieve&db=pubmed&dopt=Abstract&list_uids=6348587

- **Neurophysiological identification and characterization of thalamic neurons with single unit recording in essential tremor patients.**
  Author(s): Lee BH, Lee KH, Chung SS, Chang JW.
  Source: Acta Neurochir Suppl. 2003; 87: 133-6.
  http://www.ncbi.nlm.nih.gov/entrez/query.fcgi?cmd=Retrieve&db=pubmed&dopt=Abstract&list_uids=14518540

- **Neuropsychological and quality of life outcome after thalamic stimulation for essential tremor.**
  Author(s): Troster AI, Fields JA, Pahwa R, Wilkinson SB, Strait-Troster KA, Lyons K, Kieltyka J, Koller WC.
  Source: Neurology. 1999 November 10; 53(8): 1774-80.
  http://www.ncbi.nlm.nih.gov/entrez/query.fcgi?cmd=Retrieve&db=pubmed&dopt=Abstract&list_uids=10563627

- **Neuropsychological and quality of life outcomes 12 months after unilateral thalamic stimulation for essential tremor.**
  Author(s): Fields JA, Troster AI, Woods SP, Higginson CI, Wilkinson SB, Lyons KE, Koller WC, Pahwa R.
  Source: Journal of Neurology, Neurosurgery, and Psychiatry. 2003 March; 74(3): 305-11.
  http://www.ncbi.nlm.nih.gov/entrez/query.fcgi?cmd=Retrieve&db=pubmed&dopt=Abstract&list_uids=12588913

- **Neuropsychological deficits in essential tremor: an expression of cerebello-thalamo-cortical pathophysiology?**
  Author(s): Troster AI, Woods SP, Fields JA, Lyons KE, Pahwa R, Higginson CI, Koller WC.
  Source: European Journal of Neurology : the Official Journal of the European Federation of Neurological Societies. 2002 March; 9(2): 143-51.
  http://www.ncbi.nlm.nih.gov/entrez/query.fcgi?cmd=Retrieve&db=pubmed&dopt=Abstract&list_uids=11882055

- **Neuropsychological functioning in a patient with essential tremor with and without bilateral VIM stimulation.**
  Author(s): Lucas JA, Rippeth JD, Uitti RJ, Shuster EA, Wharen RE.
  Source: Brain and Cognition. 2000 March; 42(2): 253-67.
  http://www.ncbi.nlm.nih.gov/entrez/query.fcgi?cmd=Retrieve&db=pubmed&dopt=Abstract&list_uids=10744923

- **New alternative agents in essential tremor therapy: double-blind placebo-controlled study of alprazolam and acetazolamide.**
  Author(s): Gunal DI, Afsar N, Bekiroglu N, Aktan S.
  Source: Neurological Sciences : Official Journal of the Italian Neurological Society and of the Italian Society of Clinical Neurophysiology. 2000 October; 21(5): 315-7.
  http://www.ncbi.nlm.nih.gov/entrez/query.fcgi?cmd=Retrieve&db=pubmed&dopt=Abstract&list_uids=11286044

- **No evidence of association between CAG expansions and essential tremor in a large cohort of Italian patients.**
  Author(s): Pigullo S, Maria ED, Marchese R, Assini A, Bellone E, Scaglione C, Vitale C, Bonuccelli U, Barone P, Ajmar F, Martinelli P, Abbruzzese G, Mandich P.
  Source: Journal of Neural Transmission (Vienna, Austria : 1996). 2001; 108(3): 297-304.
  http://www.ncbi.nlm.nih.gov/entrez/query.fcgi?cmd=Retrieve&db=pubmed&dopt=Abstract&list_uids=11341481

- **Olanzapine efficacy in the treatment of essential tremor.**
  Author(s): Yetimalar Y, Irtman G, Gurgor N, Basoglu M.
  Source: European Journal of Neurology : the Official Journal of the European Federation of Neurological Societies. 2003 January; 10(1): 79-82.
  http://www.ncbi.nlm.nih.gov/entrez/query.fcgi?cmd=Retrieve&db=pubmed&dopt=Abstract&list_uids=12534999

- **Olfaction in essential tremor patients with and without isolated rest tremor.**
  Author(s): Louis ED, Jurewicz EC.
  Source: Movement Disorders : Official Journal of the Movement Disorder Society. 2003 November; 18(11): 1387-9.
  http://www.ncbi.nlm.nih.gov/entrez/query.fcgi?cmd=Retrieve&db=pubmed&dopt=Abstract&list_uids=14639689

- **Olfactory dysfunction in essential tremor: a deficit unrelated to disease duration or severity.**
  Author(s): Louis ED, Bromley SM, Jurewicz EC, Watner D.
  Source: Neurology. 2002 November 26; 59(10): 1631-3.
  http://www.ncbi.nlm.nih.gov/entrez/query.fcgi?cmd=Retrieve&db=pubmed&dopt=Abstract&list_uids=12451211

- **Olfactory function in essential tremor.**
  Author(s): Busenbark KL, Huber SJ, Greer G, Pahwa R, Koller WC.
  Source: Neurology. 1992 August; 42(8): 1631-2.
  http://www.ncbi.nlm.nih.gov/entrez/query.fcgi?cmd=Retrieve&db=pubmed&dopt=Abstract&list_uids=1641163

- **Olfactory function in essential tremor: a deficit unrelated to disease duration or severity.**
  Author(s): Hawkes C, Shah M, Findley L.
  Source: Neurology. 2003 September 23; 61(6): 871-2; Author Reply 872.
  http://www.ncbi.nlm.nih.gov/entrez/query.fcgi?cmd=Retrieve&db=pubmed&dopt=Abstract&list_uids=14504351

- **Orthostatic tremor: an association with essential tremor.**
  Author(s): FitzGerald PM, Jankovic J.
  Source: Movement Disorders : Official Journal of the Movement Disorder Society. 1991; 6(1): 60-4.
  http://www.ncbi.nlm.nih.gov/entrez/query.fcgi?cmd=Retrieve&db=pubmed&dopt=Abstract&list_uids=2005923

- **Orthostatic tremor: an essential tremor variant?**
  Author(s): Papa SM, Gershanik OS.
  Source: Movement Disorders : Official Journal of the Movement Disorder Society. 1988; 3(2): 97-108.
  http://www.ncbi.nlm.nih.gov/entrez/query.fcgi?cmd=Retrieve&db=pubmed&dopt=Abstract&list_uids=3221905

- **Orthostatic tremor: diagnostic entity or variant of essential tremor?**
  Author(s): Cleeves L, Cowan J, Findley LJ.
  Source: Journal of Neurology, Neurosurgery, and Psychiatry. 1989 January; 52(1): 130-1.
  http://www.ncbi.nlm.nih.gov/entrez/query.fcgi?cmd=Retrieve&db=pubmed&dopt=Abstract&list_uids=2709024

- **Overdiagnosis of essential tremor.**
  Author(s): Schrag A, Muenchau A, Bhatia KP, Quinn NP, Marsden CD.
  Source: Lancet. 1999 May 1; 353(9163): 1498-9.
  http://www.ncbi.nlm.nih.gov/entrez/query.fcgi?cmd=Retrieve&db=pubmed&dopt=Abstract&list_uids=10232326

- **P300 component of visual event-related potentials distinguishes patients with idiopathic parkinson's disease from patients with essential tremor.**
  Author(s): Antal A, Dibo G, Keri S, Gabor K, Janka Z, Vecsei L, Benedek G.
  Source: Journal of Neural Transmission (Vienna, Austria : 1996). 2000; 107(7): 787-97.
  http://www.ncbi.nlm.nih.gov/entrez/query.fcgi?cmd=Retrieve&db=pubmed&dopt=Abstract&list_uids=11005544

- **Parkinson's disease and essential tremor in families of patients with early-onset Parkinson's disease.**
  Author(s): Marttila RJ, Rinne UK.
  Source: Journal of Neurology, Neurosurgery, and Psychiatry. 1988 March; 51(3): 429-31.
  http://www.ncbi.nlm.nih.gov/entrez/query.fcgi?cmd=Retrieve&db=pubmed&dopt=Abstract&list_uids=3361336

- **Parkinson's disease and essential tremor.**
  Author(s): Rajput AH, Moghal S, Rajput A.
  Source: Neurology. 1994 April; 44(4): 778.
  http://www.ncbi.nlm.nih.gov/entrez/query.fcgi?cmd=Retrieve&db=pubmed&dopt=Abstract&list_uids=7695674

- **Patient education. Essential tremor.**
  Author(s): Murtagh J.
  Source: Aust Fam Physician. 1995 June; 24(6): 1125. No Abstract Available.
  http://www.ncbi.nlm.nih.gov/entrez/query.fcgi?cmd=Retrieve&db=pubmed&dopt=Abstract&list_uids=7625949

- **Peripheral silent periods in essential tremor.**
  Author(s): Shukla G, Bhatia M, Pandey RM, Behari M.
  Source: Journal of the Neurological Sciences. 2002 July 15; 199(1-2): 55-8.
  http://www.ncbi.nlm.nih.gov/entrez/query.fcgi?cmd=Retrieve&db=pubmed&dopt=Abstract&list_uids=12084443

- **Pharmacologic treatment of essential tremor.**
  Author(s): Koller WC, Hristova A, Brin M.
  Source: Neurology. 2000; 54(11 Suppl 4): S30-8. Review.
  http://www.ncbi.nlm.nih.gov/entrez/query.fcgi?cmd=Retrieve&db=pubmed&dopt=Abstract&list_uids=10854350

- **Phase resetting and frequency entrainment of essential tremor.**
  Author(s): Elble RJ, Higgins C, Hughes L.
  Source: Experimental Neurology. 1992 June; 116(3): 355-61.
  http://www.ncbi.nlm.nih.gov/entrez/query.fcgi?cmd=Retrieve&db=pubmed&dopt=Abstract&list_uids=1587336

- **Pilot trial of 1-octanol in essential tremor.**
  Author(s): Bushara KO, Goldstein SR, Grimes GJ Jr, Burstein AH, Hallett M.
  Source: Neurology. 2004 January 13; 62(1): 122-4.
  http://www.ncbi.nlm.nih.gov/entrez/query.fcgi?cmd=Retrieve&db=pubmed&dopt=Abstract&list_uids=14718713

- **Polymorphism of NACP-Rep1 in Parkinson's disease: an etiologic link with essential tremor?**
  Author(s): Tan EK, Matsuura T, Nagamitsu S, Khajavi M, Jankovic J, Ashizawa T.
  Source: Neurology. 2000 March 14; 54(5): 1195-8.
  http://www.ncbi.nlm.nih.gov/entrez/query.fcgi?cmd=Retrieve&db=pubmed&dopt=Abstract&list_uids=10720300

- **Population-based case-control study of essential tremor.**
  Author(s): Salemi G, Aridon P, Calagna G, Monte M, Savettieri G.
  Source: Italian Journal of Neurological Sciences. 1998 October; 19(5): 301-5.
  http://www.ncbi.nlm.nih.gov/entrez/query.fcgi?cmd=Retrieve&db=pubmed&dopt=Abstract&list_uids=10933450

- **Preliminary report: activation of the cerebellum in essential tremor.**
  Author(s): Colebatch JG, Findley LJ, Frackowiak RS, Marsden CD, Brooks DJ.
  Source: Lancet. 1990 October 27; 336(8722): 1028-30. Erratum In: Lancet 1990 November 24; 336(8726): 1330.
  http://www.ncbi.nlm.nih.gov/entrez/query.fcgi?cmd=Retrieve&db=pubmed&dopt=Abstract&list_uids=1977019

- **Prevalence of asymptomatic tremor in relatives of patients with essential tremor.**
  Author(s): Louis ED, Ford B, Pullman SL.
  Source: Archives of Neurology. 1997 February; 54(2): 197-200.
  http://www.ncbi.nlm.nih.gov/entrez/query.fcgi?cmd=Retrieve&db=pubmed&dopt=Abstract&list_uids=9041861

- **Prevalence of essential tremor in the Parsi community of Bombay, India.**
  Author(s): Bharucha NE, Bharucha EP, Bharucha AE, Bhise AV, Schoenberg BS.
  Source: Archives of Neurology. 1988 August; 45(8): 907-8. Erratum In: Arch Neurol 1990 January; 47(1): 11.
  http://www.ncbi.nlm.nih.gov/entrez/query.fcgi?cmd=Retrieve&db=pubmed&dopt=Abstract&list_uids=3270998

- **Prevalence of essential tremor in three elderly populations of central Spain.**
  Author(s): Benito-Leon J, Bermejo-Pareja F, Morales JM, Vega S, Molina JA.
  Source: Movement Disorders : Official Journal of the Movement Disorder Society. 2003 April; 18(4): 389-94.
  http://www.ncbi.nlm.nih.gov/entrez/query.fcgi?cmd=Retrieve&db=pubmed&dopt=Abstract&list_uids=12671944

- **Prevalence of essential tremor: a door-to-door survey in bidasoa, spain.**
  Author(s): Bergareche A, De La Puente E, Lopez De Munain A, Sarasqueta C, De Arce A, Poza JJ, Marti-Masso JF.
  Source: Neuroepidemiology. 2001 May; 20(2): 125-8.
  http://www.ncbi.nlm.nih.gov/entrez/query.fcgi?cmd=Retrieve&db=pubmed&dopt=Abstract&list_uids=11359080

- **Prevalence of essential tremor: a door-to-door survey in Terrasini, Sicily. Sicilian Neuro-Epidemiologic Study Group.**
  Author(s): Salemi G, Savettieri G, Rocca WA, Meneghini F, Saporito V, Morgante L, Reggio A, Grigoletto F, Di Perri R.
  Source: Neurology. 1994 January; 44(1): 61-4.
  http://www.ncbi.nlm.nih.gov/entrez/query.fcgi?cmd=Retrieve&db=pubmed&dopt=Abstract&list_uids=8290093

- **Prevalence of essential tremor: door-to-door neurologic exams in Mersin Province, Turkey.**
  Author(s): Dogu O, Sevim S, Camdeviren H, Sasmaz T, Bugdayci R, Aral M, Kaleagasi H, Un S, Louis ED.
  Source: Neurology. 2003 December 23; 61(12): 1804-6.
  http://www.ncbi.nlm.nih.gov/entrez/query.fcgi?cmd=Retrieve&db=pubmed&dopt=Abstract&list_uids=14694055

- **Primidone in the long-term treatment of essential tremor: a prospective study with computerized quantitative analysis.**
  Author(s): Sasso E, Perucca E, Fava R, Calzetti S.
  Source: Clinical Neuropharmacology. 1990 February; 13(1): 67-76.
  http://www.ncbi.nlm.nih.gov/entrez/query.fcgi?cmd=Retrieve&db=pubmed&dopt=Abstract&list_uids=2306749

- **Propranolol, clonidine, urapidil and trazodone infusion in essential tremor: a double-blind crossover trial.**
  Author(s): Caccia MR, Osio M, Galimberti V, Cataldi G, Mangoni A.
  Source: Acta Neurologica Scandinavica. 1989 May; 79(5): 379-83.
  http://www.ncbi.nlm.nih.gov/entrez/query.fcgi?cmd=Retrieve&db=pubmed&dopt=Abstract&list_uids=2741669

- **Pulse width is associated with cognitive decline after thalamic stimulation for essential tremor.**
  Author(s): Woods SP, Fields JA, Lyons KE, Pahwa R, Troster AI.
  Source: Parkinsonism & Related Disorders. 2003 June; 9(5): 295-300.
  http://www.ncbi.nlm.nih.gov/entrez/query.fcgi?cmd=Retrieve&db=pubmed&dopt=Abstract&list_uids=12781597

- **Quantification of essential tremor in writing and drawing.**
  Author(s): Elble RJ, Brilliant M, Leffler K, Higgins C.
  Source: Movement Disorders : Official Journal of the Movement Disorder Society. 1996 January; 11(1): 70-8.
  http://www.ncbi.nlm.nih.gov/entrez/query.fcgi?cmd=Retrieve&db=pubmed&dopt=Abstract&list_uids=8771070

- **Quantitative assessment of parkinsonian and essential tremor: clinical application of triaxial accelerometry.**
  Author(s): Jankovic J, Frost JD Jr.
  Source: Neurology. 1981 October; 31(10): 1235-40.
  http://www.ncbi.nlm.nih.gov/entrez/query.fcgi?cmd=Retrieve&db=pubmed&dopt=Abstract&list_uids=7202133

- **Quetiapine and essential tremor.**
  Author(s): Micheli F, Cersosimo MG, Raina G, Gatto E.
  Source: Clinical Neuropharmacology. 2002 November-December; 25(6): 303-6.
  http://www.ncbi.nlm.nih.gov/entrez/query.fcgi?cmd=Retrieve&db=pubmed&dopt=Abstract&list_uids=12469002

- **Randomized trial comparing primidone initiation schedules for treating essential tremor.**
  Author(s): O'Suilleabhain P, Dewey RB Jr.
  Source: Movement Disorders : Official Journal of the Movement Disorder Society. 2002 March; 17(2): 382-6.
  http://www.ncbi.nlm.nih.gov/entrez/query.fcgi?cmd=Retrieve&db=pubmed&dopt=Abstract&list_uids=11921128

- **Rapid wrist movements in patients with essential tremor. The critical role of the second agonist burst.**
  Author(s): Britton TC, Thompson PD, Day BL, Rothwell JC, Findley LJ, Marsden CD.
  Source: Brain; a Journal of Neurology. 1994 February; 117 (Pt 1): 39-47.
  http://www.ncbi.nlm.nih.gov/entrez/query.fcgi?cmd=Retrieve&db=pubmed&dopt=Abstract&list_uids=8149213

- **Reciprocal inhibition in forearm muscles in patients with essential tremor.**
  Author(s): Mercuri B, Berardelli A, Modugno N, Vacca L, Ruggieri S, Manfredi M.
  Source: Muscle & Nerve. 1998 June; 21(6): 796-9.
  http://www.ncbi.nlm.nih.gov/entrez/query.fcgi?cmd=Retrieve&db=pubmed&dopt=Abstract&list_uids=9585335

- **Red nuclear and cerebellar but no olivary activation associated with essential tremor: a positron emission tomographic study.**
  Author(s): Wills AJ, Jenkins IH, Thompson PD, Findley LJ, Brooks DJ.
  Source: Annals of Neurology. 1994 October; 36(4): 636-42.
  http://www.ncbi.nlm.nih.gov/entrez/query.fcgi?cmd=Retrieve&db=pubmed&dopt=Abstract&list_uids=7944296

- **Reduced body mass index in patients with essential tremor: a population-based study in the province of Mersin, Turkey.**
  Author(s): Dogu O, Sevim S, Louis ED, Kaleagasi H, Aral M.
  Source: Archives of Neurology. 2004 March; 61(3): 386-9.
  http://www.ncbi.nlm.nih.gov/entrez/query.fcgi?cmd=Retrieve&db=pubmed&dopt=Abstract&list_uids=15023816

- **Regional and racial differences in the prevalence of physician-diagnosed essential tremor in the United States.**
  Author(s): Louis ED, Fried LP, Fitzpatrick AL, Longstreth WT Jr, Newman AB.
  Source: Movement Disorders : Official Journal of the Movement Disorder Society. 2003 September; 18(9): 1035-40.
  http://www.ncbi.nlm.nih.gov/entrez/query.fcgi?cmd=Retrieve&db=pubmed&dopt=Abstract&list_uids=14502671

- **Relationship between plasma propranolol concentration and relief of essential tremor.**
  Author(s): Jefferson D, Jenner P, Marsden CD.
  Source: Journal of Neurology, Neurosurgery, and Psychiatry. 1979 September; 42(9): 831-7.
  http://www.ncbi.nlm.nih.gov/entrez/query.fcgi?cmd=Retrieve&db=pubmed&dopt=Abstract&list_uids=501384

- **Reliability between two observers using a protocol for diagnosing essential tremor.**
  Author(s): Louis ED, Ford B, Bismuth B.
  Source: Movement Disorders : Official Journal of the Movement Disorder Society. 1998 March; 13(2): 287-93.
  http://www.ncbi.nlm.nih.gov/entrez/query.fcgi?cmd=Retrieve&db=pubmed&dopt=Abstract&list_uids=9539343

- **Report on the effects of introducing primidone for essential tremor.**
  Author(s): Porter RM.
  Source: The Medical Journal of Australia. 1992 December 7-21; 157(11-12): 840, 842.
  http://www.ncbi.nlm.nih.gov/entrez/query.fcgi?cmd=Retrieve&db=pubmed&dopt=Abstract&list_uids=1454027

- **Resetting of essential tremor and postural tremor in Parkinson's disease with transcranial magnetic stimulation.**
  Author(s): Pascual-Leone A, Valls-Sole J, Toro C, Wassermann EM, Hallett M.
  Source: Muscle & Nerve. 1994 July; 17(7): 800-7.
  http://www.ncbi.nlm.nih.gov/entrez/query.fcgi?cmd=Retrieve&db=pubmed&dopt=Abstract&list_uids=8008009

- **Resetting of tremor by mechanical perturbations: a comparison of essential tremor and parkinsonian tremor.**
  Author(s): Lee RG, Stein RB.
  Source: Annals of Neurology. 1981 December; 10(6): 523-31.
  http://www.ncbi.nlm.nih.gov/entrez/query.fcgi?cmd=Retrieve&db=pubmed&dopt=Abstract&list_uids=7325601

- **Rest tremor in patients with essential tremor: prevalence, clinical correlates, and electrophysiologic characteristics.**
  Author(s): Cohen O, Pullman S, Jurewicz E, Watner D, Louis ED.
  Source: Archives of Neurology. 2003 March; 60(3): 405-10.
  http://www.ncbi.nlm.nih.gov/entrez/query.fcgi?cmd=Retrieve&db=pubmed&dopt=Abstract&list_uids=12633153

- **Resting tremor only: a variant of Parkinson's disease or of essential tremor.**
  Author(s): Chang MH, Chang TW, Lai PH, Sy CG.
  Source: Journal of the Neurological Sciences. 1995 June; 130(2): 215-9.
  http://www.ncbi.nlm.nih.gov/entrez/query.fcgi?cmd=Retrieve&db=pubmed&dopt=Abstract&list_uids=8586989

- **Risk of tremor and impairment from tremor in relatives of patients with essential tremor: a community-based family study.**
  Author(s): Louis ED, Ford B, Frucht S, Barnes LF, X-Tang M, Ottman R.
  Source: Annals of Neurology. 2001 June; 49(6): 761-9.
  http://www.ncbi.nlm.nih.gov/entrez/query.fcgi?cmd=Retrieve&db=pubmed&dopt=Abstract&list_uids=11409428

- **Selective adrenergic beta-2-receptor blocking drug, ICI-118.551, is effective in essential tremor.**
  Author(s): Teravainen H, Huttunen J, Larsen TA.
  Source: Acta Neurologica Scandinavica. 1986 July; 74(1): 34-7.
  http://www.ncbi.nlm.nih.gov/entrez/query.fcgi?cmd=Retrieve&db=pubmed&dopt=Abstract&list_uids=2876576

- **Selective disappearance of essential tremor after ischaemic stroke.**
  Author(s): Le Pira F, Giuffrida S, Panetta MR, Lo Bartolo ML, Politi G.
  Source: European Journal of Neurology : the Official Journal of the European Federation of Neurological Societies. 2004 June; 11(6): 422-3.
  http://www.ncbi.nlm.nih.gov/entrez/query.fcgi?cmd=Retrieve&db=pubmed&dopt=Abstract&list_uids=15171740

- **Severe essential tremor compared with Parkinson's disease in male veterans: diagnostic characteristics, treatment, and psychosocial complications.**
  Author(s): Metzer WS.
  Source: Southern Medical Journal. 1992 August; 85(8): 825-8.
  http://www.ncbi.nlm.nih.gov/entrez/query.fcgi?cmd=Retrieve&db=pubmed&dopt=Abstract&list_uids=1502624

- **Severe upper airway obstruction in essential tremor presenting as asthma.**
  Author(s): Izquierdo-Alonso JL, Martinez-Martin P, Juretschke-Moragues MA, Serrano-Iglesias JA.
  Source: The European Respiratory Journal : Official Journal of the European Society for Clinical Respiratory Physiology. 1994 June; 7(6): 1182-4.
  http://www.ncbi.nlm.nih.gov/entrez/query.fcgi?cmd=Retrieve&db=pubmed&dopt=Abstract&list_uids=7925890

- **Significance of parkinsonian manifestations in essential tremor.**
  Author(s): Rajput AH, Rozdilsky B, Ang L, Rajput A.
  Source: The Canadian Journal of Neurological Sciences. Le Journal Canadien Des Sciences Neurologiques. 1993 May; 20(2): 114-7.
  http://www.ncbi.nlm.nih.gov/entrez/query.fcgi?cmd=Retrieve&db=pubmed&dopt=Abstract&list_uids=8334571

- **Skin color and the risk and severity of essential tremor: a reflectance spectroscopy study.**
  Author(s): Louis ED, Jurewicz EC, Watner D, Factor-Litvak P.
  Source: Parkinsonism & Related Disorders. 2003 March; 9(4): 239-41.
  http://www.ncbi.nlm.nih.gov/entrez/query.fcgi?cmd=Retrieve&db=pubmed&dopt=Abstract&list_uids=12618060

- **Social phobia secondary to physical disability. A review of benign essential tremor (BET) and stuttering.**
  Author(s): George MS, Lydiard RB.
  Source: Psychosomatics. 1994 November-December; 35(6): 520-3. Review.
  http://www.ncbi.nlm.nih.gov/entrez/query.fcgi?cmd=Retrieve&db=pubmed&dopt=A
  bstract&list_uids=7809354

- **Specificity of ethanol in essential tremor.**
  Author(s): Rajput AH.
  Source: Annals of Neurology. 1996 December; 40(6): 950-1.
  http://www.ncbi.nlm.nih.gov/entrez/query.fcgi?cmd=Retrieve&db=pubmed&dopt=A
  bstract&list_uids=9007108

- **Spectral electromyographic analysis of essential tremor.**
  Author(s): Ivanova-Smolenskaya IA, Kandel' EI, Andreeva EA, Smirnova SN, Khutorskaya OE.
  Source: Neuroscience and Behavioral Physiology. 1987 November-December; 17(6): 513-8.
  http://www.ncbi.nlm.nih.gov/entrez/query.fcgi?cmd=Retrieve&db=pubmed&dopt=A
  bstract&list_uids=3441283

- **Stereotactic thalamotomy for medically intractable essential tremor.**
  Author(s): Goldman MS, Kelly PJ.
  Source: Stereotactic and Functional Neurosurgery. 1992; 58(1-4): 22-5.
  http://www.ncbi.nlm.nih.gov/entrez/query.fcgi?cmd=Retrieve&db=pubmed&dopt=A
  bstract&list_uids=1439342

- **Stereotactic thalamotomy in the treatment of essential tremor of the upper extremity: reassessment including a blinded measure of outcome.**
  Author(s): Zirh A, Reich SG, Dougherty PM, Lenz FA.
  Source: Journal of Neurology, Neurosurgery, and Psychiatry. 1999 June; 66(6): 772-5.
  http://www.ncbi.nlm.nih.gov/entrez/query.fcgi?cmd=Retrieve&db=pubmed&dopt=A
  bstract&list_uids=10329753

- **Stereotactic ventral intermedial thalamotomy for the treatment of essential tremor: results of a series of 37 patients.**
  Author(s): Akbostanci MC, Slavin KV, Burchiel KJ.
  Source: Stereotactic and Functional Neurosurgery. 1999; 72(2-4): 174-7.
  http://www.ncbi.nlm.nih.gov/entrez/query.fcgi?cmd=Retrieve&db=pubmed&dopt=A
  bstract&list_uids=10853074

- **Stimulation of the ventral intermediate thalamic nucleus in tremor dominated Parkinson's disease and essential tremor.**
  Author(s): Alesch F, Pinter MM, Helscher RJ, Fertl L, Benabid AL, Koos WT.
  Source: Acta Neurochirurgica. 1995; 136(1-2): 75-81.
  http://www.ncbi.nlm.nih.gov/entrez/query.fcgi?cmd=Retrieve&db=pubmed&dopt=A
  bstract&list_uids=8748831

- **Strength training can improve steadiness in persons with essential tremor.**
  Author(s): Bilodeau M, Keen DA, Sweeney PJ, Shields RW, Enoka RM.
  Source: Muscle & Nerve. 2000 May; 23(5): 771-8.
  http://www.ncbi.nlm.nih.gov/entrez/query.fcgi?cmd=Retrieve&db=pubmed&dopt=A
  bstract&list_uids=10797401

- **Stretch reflex oscillations and essential tremor.**
  Author(s): Elble RJ, Higgins C, Moody CJ.
  Source: Journal of Neurology, Neurosurgery, and Psychiatry. 1987 June; 50(6): 691-8.
  http://www.ncbi.nlm.nih.gov/entrez/query.fcgi?cmd=Retrieve&db=pubmed&dopt=A
  bstract&list_uids=3612149

- **Subdivision of essential tremor patients according to physiologic characteristics.**
  Author(s): Golan D, Giladi N, Thorne R, Korczyn AD, Simon ES.
  Source: Acta Neurologica Scandinavica. 2004 June; 109(6): 393-7.
  http://www.ncbi.nlm.nih.gov/entrez/query.fcgi?cmd=Retrieve&db=pubmed&dopt=A
  bstract&list_uids=15147462

- **Surgical interventions in the treatment of Parkinson's disease (PD) and essential tremor (ET): medial pallidotomy in PD and chronic deep brain stimulation (DBS) in PD and ET.**
  Author(s): Duff J, Sime E.
  Source: Axone. 1997 June; 18(4): 85-9.
  http://www.ncbi.nlm.nih.gov/entrez/query.fcgi?cmd=Retrieve&db=pubmed&dopt=A
  bstract&list_uids=9295483

- **Surgical treatment of essential tremor.**
  Author(s): Pahwa R, Lyons K, Koller WC.
  Source: Neurology. 2000; 54(11 Suppl 4): S39-44. Review.
  http://www.ncbi.nlm.nih.gov/entrez/query.fcgi?cmd=Retrieve&db=pubmed&dopt=A
  bstract&list_uids=10854351

- **Survey of essential tremor patients on their knowledge about the genetics of the disease.**
  Author(s): Watner D, Jurewicz EC, Louis ED.
  Source: Movement Disorders : Official Journal of the Movement Disorder Society. 2002 March; 17(2): 378-81.
  http://www.ncbi.nlm.nih.gov/entrez/query.fcgi?cmd=Retrieve&db=pubmed&dopt=A
  bstract&list_uids=11921127

- **Test-retest reliability of patient information on age of onset in essential tremor.**
  Author(s): Louis ED, Schonberger RB, Parides M, Ford B, Barnes LF.
  Source: Movement Disorders : Official Journal of the Movement Disorder Society. 2000 July; 15(4): 738-41.
  http://www.ncbi.nlm.nih.gov/entrez/query.fcgi?cmd=Retrieve&db=pubmed&dopt=A
  bstract&list_uids=10928590

- **Thalamic neuronal activity correlated with essential tremor.**
  Author(s): Hua SE, Lenz FA, Zirh TA, Reich SG, Dougherty PM.
  Source: Journal of Neurology, Neurosurgery, and Psychiatry. 1998 February; 64(2): 273-6.
  http://www.ncbi.nlm.nih.gov/entrez/query.fcgi?cmd=Retrieve&db=pubmed&dopt=Abstract&list_uids=9489548

- **Thalamic stimulation for essential tremor activates motor and deactivates vestibular cortex.**
  Author(s): Ceballos-Baumann AO, Boecker H, Fogel W, Alesch F, Bartenstein P, Conrad B, Diederich N, von Falkenhayn I, Moringlane JR, Schwaiger M, Tronnier VM.
  Source: Neurology. 2001 May 22; 56(10): 1347-54.
  http://www.ncbi.nlm.nih.gov/entrez/query.fcgi?cmd=Retrieve&db=pubmed&dopt=Abstract&list_uids=11376186

- **Thalamic stimulation for the treatment of midline tremors in essential tremor patients.**
  Author(s): Obwegeser AA, Uitti RJ, Turk MF, Strongosky AJ, Wharen RE.
  Source: Neurology. 2000 June 27; 54(12): 2342-4.
  http://www.ncbi.nlm.nih.gov/entrez/query.fcgi?cmd=Retrieve&db=pubmed&dopt=Abstract&list_uids=10881269

- **Thalamic stimulation in essential tremor.**
  Author(s): Limousin-Dowsey P.
  Source: Lancet. Neurology. 2004 February; 3(2): 80. Review.
  http://www.ncbi.nlm.nih.gov/entrez/query.fcgi?cmd=Retrieve&db=pubmed&dopt=Abstract&list_uids=14746995

- **Thalamic stimulation reduces essential tremor but not the delayed antagonist muscle timing.**
  Author(s): Zackowski KM, Bastian AJ, Hakimian S, Mink JW, Perlmutter JS, Koller WC, Thach WT Jr.
  Source: Neurology. 2002 February 12; 58(3): 402-10.
  http://www.ncbi.nlm.nih.gov/entrez/query.fcgi?cmd=Retrieve&db=pubmed&dopt=Abstract&list_uids=11839839

- **The cerebellothalamocortical pathway in essential tremor.**
  Author(s): Pinto AD, Lang AE, Chen R.
  Source: Neurology. 2003 June 24; 60(12): 1985-7.
  http://www.ncbi.nlm.nih.gov/entrez/query.fcgi?cmd=Retrieve&db=pubmed&dopt=Abstract&list_uids=12821747

- **The contribution of tremor studies to diagnosis of parkinsonian and essential tremor: a statistical evaluation.**
  Author(s): Burne JA, Hayes MW, Fung VS, Yiannikas C, Boljevac D.
  Source: Journal of Clinical Neuroscience : Official Journal of the Neurosurgical Society of Australasia. 2002 May; 9(3): 237-42.
  http://www.ncbi.nlm.nih.gov/entrez/query.fcgi?cmd=Retrieve&db=pubmed&dopt=Abstract&list_uids=12093126

- **The fragile X premutation presenting as essential tremor.**
  Author(s): Leehey MA, Munhoz RP, Lang AE, Brunberg JA, Grigsby J, Greco C, Jacquemont S, Tassone F, Lozano AM, Hagerman PJ, Hagerman RJ.
  Source: Archives of Neurology. 2003 January; 60(1): 117-21.
  http://www.ncbi.nlm.nih.gov/entrez/query.fcgi?cmd=Retrieve&db=pubmed&dopt=Abstract&list_uids=12533098

- **The gait disorder of advanced essential tremor.**
  Author(s): Stolze H, Petersen G, Raethjen J, Wenzelburger R, Deuschl G.
  Source: Brain; a Journal of Neurology. 2001 November; 124(Pt 11): 2278-86.
  http://www.ncbi.nlm.nih.gov/entrez/query.fcgi?cmd=Retrieve&db=pubmed&dopt=Abstract&list_uids=11673328

- **The impact of thalamic stimulation on activities of daily living for essential tremor.**
  Author(s): Bryant JA, De Salles A, Cabatan C, Frysinger R, Behnke E, Bronstein J.
  Source: Surgical Neurology. 2003 June; 59(6): 479-84; Discussion 484-5.
  http://www.ncbi.nlm.nih.gov/entrez/query.fcgi?cmd=Retrieve&db=pubmed&dopt=Abstract&list_uids=12826348

- **The pathophysiology of essential tremor.**
  Author(s): Deuschl G, Elble RJ.
  Source: Neurology. 2000; 54(11 Suppl 4): S14-20. Review.
  http://www.ncbi.nlm.nih.gov/entrez/query.fcgi?cmd=Retrieve&db=pubmed&dopt=Abstract&list_uids=10854347

- **The Washington Heights-Inwood Genetic Study of Essential Tremor: methodologic issues in essential-tremor research.**
  Author(s): Louis ED, Ottman R, Ford B, Pullman S, Martinez M, Fahn S, Hauser WA.
  Source: Neuroepidemiology. 1997; 16(3): 124-33.
  http://www.ncbi.nlm.nih.gov/entrez/query.fcgi?cmd=Retrieve&db=pubmed&dopt=Abstract&list_uids=9159767

- **Three-dimensional measurement of essential tremor.**
  Author(s): Matsumoto JY, Dodick DW, Stevens LN, Newman RC, Caskey PE, Fjerstad W.
  Source: Movement Disorders : Official Journal of the Movement Disorder Society. 1999 March; 14(2): 288-94.
  http://www.ncbi.nlm.nih.gov/entrez/query.fcgi?cmd=Retrieve&db=pubmed&dopt=Abstract&list_uids=10091623

- **Tolerance and tremor rebound following long-term chronic thalamic stimulation for Parkinsonian and essential tremor.**
  Author(s): Hariz MI, Shamsgovara P, Johansson F, Hariz G, Fodstad H.
  Source: Stereotactic and Functional Neurosurgery. 1999; 72(2-4): 208-18.
  http://www.ncbi.nlm.nih.gov/entrez/query.fcgi?cmd=Retrieve&db=pubmed&dopt=Abstract&list_uids=10853080

- **Topiramate and essential tremor.**
  Author(s): Galvez-Jimenez N, Hargreave M.
  Source: Annals of Neurology. 2000 June; 47(6): 837-8.
  http://www.ncbi.nlm.nih.gov/entrez/query.fcgi?cmd=Retrieve&db=pubmed&dopt=A
  bstract&list_uids=10852557

- **Tremor arrest with thalamic microinjections of muscimol in patients with essential tremor.**
  Author(s): Pahapill PA, Levy R, Dostrovsky JO, Davis KD, Rezai AR, Tasker RR, Lozano AM.
  Source: Annals of Neurology. 1999 August; 46(2): 249-52.
  http://www.ncbi.nlm.nih.gov/entrez/query.fcgi?cmd=Retrieve&db=pubmed&dopt=A
  bstract&list_uids=10443891

- **Tremor frequency patterns in mercury vapor exposure, compared with early Parkinson's disease and essential tremor.**
  Author(s): Biernat H, Ellias SA, Wermuth L, Cleary D, de Oliveira Santos EC, Jorgensen PJ, Feldman RG, Grandjean P.
  Source: Neurotoxicology. 1999 December; 20(6): 945-52.
  http://www.ncbi.nlm.nih.gov/entrez/query.fcgi?cmd=Retrieve&db=pubmed&dopt=A
  bstract&list_uids=10693975

- **Tremor-correlated cortical activity in essential tremor.**
  Author(s): Hellwig B, Haussler S, Schelter B, Lauk M, Guschlbauer B, Timmer J, Lucking CH.
  Source: Lancet. 2001 February 17; 357(9255): 519-23.
  http://www.ncbi.nlm.nih.gov/entrez/query.fcgi?cmd=Retrieve&db=pubmed&dopt=A
  bstract&list_uids=11229671

- **Understanding essential tremor. Differential diagnosis and options for treatment.**
  Author(s): Evidente VG.
  Source: Postgraduate Medicine. 2000 October; 108(5): 138-40, 143-6, 149. Review.
  http://www.ncbi.nlm.nih.gov/entrez/query.fcgi?cmd=Retrieve&db=pubmed&dopt=A
  bstract&list_uids=11043086

- **Unilateral disappearance of essential tremor after cerebral hemispheric infarct.**
  Author(s): Constantino AE, Louis ED.
  Source: Journal of Neurology. 2003 March; 250(3): 354-5.
  http://www.ncbi.nlm.nih.gov/entrez/query.fcgi?cmd=Retrieve&db=pubmed&dopt=A
  bstract&list_uids=12749318

- **Unilateral essential tremor after wrist immobilization: a case report.**
  Author(s): Cole JD, Illis LS, Sedgwick EM.
  Source: Journal of Neurology, Neurosurgery, and Psychiatry. 1989 February; 52(2): 286-7.
  http://www.ncbi.nlm.nih.gov/entrez/query.fcgi?cmd=Retrieve&db=pubmed&dopt=A
  bstract&list_uids=2703848

- **Unilateral thalamic deep brain stimulation for refractory essential tremor and Parkinson's disease tremor.**
  Author(s): Ondo W, Jankovic J, Schwartz K, Almaguer M, Simpson RK.
  Source: Neurology. 1998 October; 51(4): 1063-9.
  http://www.ncbi.nlm.nih.gov/entrez/query.fcgi?cmd=Retrieve&db=pubmed&dopt=Abstract&list_uids=9781530

- **Unusual motor conduction velocity values in Charcot-Marie-Tooth disease associated with essential tremor: report of a kinship.**
  Author(s): Salisachs P.
  Source: European Neurology. 1975; 13(4): 377-82.
  http://www.ncbi.nlm.nih.gov/entrez/query.fcgi?cmd=Retrieve&db=pubmed&dopt=Abstract&list_uids=1149757

- **Use of primidone in low doses (250 mg/day) versus high doses (750 mg/day) in the management of essential tremor. Double-blind comparative study with one-year follow-up.**
  Author(s): Serrano-Duenas M.
  Source: Parkinsonism & Related Disorders. 2003 October; 10(1): 29-33.
  http://www.ncbi.nlm.nih.gov/entrez/query.fcgi?cmd=Retrieve&db=pubmed&dopt=Abstract&list_uids=14499204

- **Vagus nerve stimulation for essential tremor: a pilot efficacy and safety trial.**
  Author(s): Handforth A, Ondo WG, Tatter S, Mathern GW, Simpson RK Jr, Walker F, Sutton JP, Hubble JP, Jankovic J.
  Source: Neurology. 2003 November 25; 61(10): 1401-5.
  http://www.ncbi.nlm.nih.gov/entrez/query.fcgi?cmd=Retrieve&db=pubmed&dopt=Abstract&list_uids=14638963

- **Validity and test-retest reliability of a disability questionnaire for essential tremor.**
  Author(s): Louis ED, Barnes LF, Wendt KJ, Albert SM, Pullman SL, Yu Q, Schneier FR.
  Source: Movement Disorders : Official Journal of the Movement Disorder Society. 2000 May; 15(3): 516-23.
  http://www.ncbi.nlm.nih.gov/entrez/query.fcgi?cmd=Retrieve&db=pubmed&dopt=Abstract&list_uids=10830418

- **Validity of a performance-based test of function in essential tremor.**
  Author(s): Louis ED, Wendt KJ, Albert SM, Pullman SL, Yu Q, Andrews H.
  Source: Archives of Neurology. 1999 July; 56(7): 841-6.
  http://www.ncbi.nlm.nih.gov/entrez/query.fcgi?cmd=Retrieve&db=pubmed&dopt=Abstract&list_uids=10404986

- **Validity of family history data on essential tremor.**
  Author(s): Louis ED, Ford B, Wendt KJ, Ottman R.
  Source: Movement Disorders : Official Journal of the Movement Disorder Society. 1999 May; 14(3): 456-61.
  http://www.ncbi.nlm.nih.gov/entrez/query.fcgi?cmd=Retrieve&db=pubmed&dopt=Abstract&list_uids=10348469

- **Variability in amplitude of untreated essential tremor.**
  Author(s): Cleeves L, Findley LJ.
  Source: Journal of Neurology, Neurosurgery, and Psychiatry. 1987 June; 50(6): 704-8.
  http://www.ncbi.nlm.nih.gov/entrez/query.fcgi?cmd=Retrieve&db=pubmed&dopt=Abstract&list_uids=3612150

- **Visuomotor performance in patients with essential tremor.**
  Author(s): Schwartz M, Badarny S, Gofman S, Hocherman S.
  Source: Movement Disorders : Official Journal of the Movement Disorder Society. 1999 November; 14(6): 988-93.
  http://www.ncbi.nlm.nih.gov/entrez/query.fcgi?cmd=Retrieve&db=pubmed&dopt=Abstract&list_uids=10584674

- **Writing tremor: its relationship to benign essential tremor.**
  Author(s): Kachi T, Rothwell JC, Cowan JM, Marsden CD.
  Source: Journal of Neurology, Neurosurgery, and Psychiatry. 1985 June; 48(6): 545-50.
  http://www.ncbi.nlm.nih.gov/entrez/query.fcgi?cmd=Retrieve&db=pubmed&dopt=Abstract&list_uids=4009190

- **Writing tremor: its relationship to essential tremor.**
  Author(s): Koller WC, Martyn B.
  Source: Journal of Neurology, Neurosurgery, and Psychiatry. 1986 February; 49(2): 220.
  http://www.ncbi.nlm.nih.gov/entrez/query.fcgi?cmd=Retrieve&db=pubmed&dopt=Abstract&list_uids=3950645

CHAPTER 2. ALTERNATIVE MEDICINE AND ESSENTIAL TREMOR

Overview

In this chapter, we will begin by introducing you to official information sources on complementary and alternative medicine (CAM) relating to essential tremor. At the conclusion of this chapter, we will provide additional sources.

National Center for Complementary and Alternative Medicine

The National Center for Complementary and Alternative Medicine (NCCAM) of the National Institutes of Health (**http://nccam.nih.gov/**) has created a link to the National Library of Medicine's databases to facilitate research for articles that specifically relate to essential tremor and complementary medicine. To search the database, go to the following Web site: **http://www.nlm.nih.gov/nccam/camonpubmed.html**. Select "CAM on PubMed." Enter "essential tremor" (or synonyms) into the search box. Click "Go." The following references provide information on particular aspects of complementary and alternative medicine that are related to essential tremor:

- **Acute effect of transcutaneous electrical nerve stimulation on tremor.**
  Author(s): Munhoz RP, Hanajima R, Ashby P, Lang AE.
  Source: Movement Disorders : Official Journal of the Movement Disorder Society. 2003 February; 18(2): 191-4.
  http://www.ncbi.nlm.nih.gov/entrez/query.fcgi?cmd=Retrieve&db=pubmed&dopt=Abstract&list_uids=12539214

- **Application of 5 HTP in the treatment of essential tremor.**
  Author(s): Guillard A, Chastang C.
  Source: Int J Neurol. 1979; 13(1-4): 251-3. No Abstract Available.
  http://www.ncbi.nlm.nih.gov/entrez/query.fcgi?cmd=Retrieve&db=pubmed&dopt=Abstract&list_uids=318090

- **Applications of transcranial magnetic stimulation in movement disorders.**
  Author(s): Cantello R.

Source: Journal of Clinical Neurophysiology : Official Publication of the American Electroencephalographic Society. 2002 August; 19(4): 272-93. Review.
http://www.ncbi.nlm.nih.gov/entrez/query.fcgi?cmd=Retrieve&db=pubmed&dopt=Abstract&list_uids=12436085

- **Behavioral relaxation training for tremor disorders in older adults.**
  Author(s): Chung W, Poppen R, Lundervold DA.
  Source: Biofeedback Self Regul. 1995 June; 20(2): 123-35.
  http://www.ncbi.nlm.nih.gov/entrez/query.fcgi?cmd=Retrieve&db=pubmed&dopt=Abstract&list_uids=7662749

- **Biobehavioral intervention for older adults coping with essential tremor.**
  Author(s): Lundervold DA, Poppen R.
  Source: Applied Psychophysiology and Biofeedback. 2004 March; 29(1): 63-73.
  http://www.ncbi.nlm.nih.gov/entrez/query.fcgi?cmd=Retrieve&db=pubmed&dopt=Abstract&list_uids=15077465

- **Biobehavioral rehabilitation for older adults with essential tremor.**
  Author(s): Lundervold DA, Poppen R.
  Source: The Gerontologist. 1995 August; 35(4): 556-9.
  http://www.ncbi.nlm.nih.gov/entrez/query.fcgi?cmd=Retrieve&db=pubmed&dopt=Abstract&list_uids=7557528

- **Cutaneous electrosurgery in a patient with a deep brain stimulator.**
  Author(s): Weaver J, Kim SJ, Lee MH, Torres A.
  Source: Dermatologic Surgery : Official Publication for American Society for Dermatologic Surgery [et Al.]. 1999 May; 25(5): 415-7. Erratum In: Dermatol Surg 1999 October; 25(10): 829.
  http://www.ncbi.nlm.nih.gov/entrez/query.fcgi?cmd=Retrieve&db=pubmed&dopt=Abstract&list_uids=10469084

- **Life-threatening parkinsonism induced by kava-kava.**
  Author(s): Meseguer E, Taboada R, Sanchez V, Mena MA, Campos V, Garcia De Yebenes J.
  Source: Movement Disorders : Official Journal of the Movement Disorder Society. 2002 January; 17(1): 195-6.
  http://www.ncbi.nlm.nih.gov/entrez/query.fcgi?cmd=Retrieve&db=pubmed&dopt=Abstract&list_uids=11835463

- **Management of essential tremor.**
  Author(s): Zesiewicz TA, Encarnacion E, Hauser RA.
  Source: Curr Neurol Neurosci Rep. 2002 July; 2(4): 324-30. Review.
  http://www.ncbi.nlm.nih.gov/entrez/query.fcgi?cmd=Retrieve&db=pubmed&dopt=Abstract&list_uids=12044252

- **New approaches in the management of hyperkinetic movement disorders.**
  Author(s): Fahn S.

Source: Advances in Experimental Medicine and Biology. 1977; 90: 157-73.
http://www.ncbi.nlm.nih.gov/entrez/query.fcgi?cmd=Retrieve&db=pubmed&dopt=A
bstract&list_uids=303860

- **Psychophysiologic test performance in normal twins and in a pair of identical twins with essential tremor that is suppressed by alcohol.**
  Author(s): Propping P.
  Source: Human Genetics. 1977 May 10; 36(3): 321-5.
  http://www.ncbi.nlm.nih.gov/entrez/query.fcgi?cmd=Retrieve&db=pubmed&dopt=A
  bstract&list_uids=558152

- **Reduction of tremor severity and disability following behavioral relaxation training.**
  Author(s): Lundervold DA, Belwood MF, Craney JL, Poppen R.
  Source: Journal of Behavior Therapy and Experimental Psychiatry. 1999 June; 30(2): 119-35.
  http://www.ncbi.nlm.nih.gov/entrez/query.fcgi?cmd=Retrieve&db=pubmed&dopt=A
  bstract&list_uids=10489088

- **Single-pulse transcranial magnetic stimulation reset the rhythm of essential tremor but not heart beat.**
  Author(s): Yu HY, Chen JT, Lee YC, Guo YC, Kao CD, Shan DE, Liao KK.
  Source: Zhonghua Yi Xue Za Zhi (Taipei). 2001 May; 64(5): 271-6.
  http://www.ncbi.nlm.nih.gov/entrez/query.fcgi?cmd=Retrieve&db=pubmed&dopt=A
  bstract&list_uids=11499336

- **Transcranial magnetic stimulation of the cerebellum in essential tremor: a controlled study.**
  Author(s): Gironell A, Kulisevsky J, Lorenzo J, Barbanoj M, Pascual-Sedano B, Otermin P.
  Source: Archives of Neurology. 2002 March; 59(3): 413-7.
  http://www.ncbi.nlm.nih.gov/entrez/query.fcgi?cmd=Retrieve&db=pubmed&dopt=A
  bstract&list_uids=11890845

- **Treatment of lithium-induced tremor and familial essential tremor with essential fatty acids.**
  Author(s): Lieb J, Horrobin DF.
  Source: Progress in Lipid Research. 1981; 20: 535-7.
  http://www.ncbi.nlm.nih.gov/entrez/query.fcgi?cmd=Retrieve&db=pubmed&dopt=A
  bstract&list_uids=7342107

- **Tremor response to polarity, voltage, pulsewidth and frequency of thalamic stimulation.**
  Author(s): O'Suilleabhain PE, Frawley W, Giller C, Dewey RB Jr.
  Source: Neurology. 2003 March 11; 60(5): 786-90.
  http://www.ncbi.nlm.nih.gov/entrez/query.fcgi?cmd=Retrieve&db=pubmed&dopt=A
  bstract&list_uids=12629234

Additional Web Resources

A number of additional Web sites offer encyclopedic information covering CAM and related topics. The following is a representative sample:

- Alternative Medicine Foundation, Inc.: **http://www.herbmed.org/**
- AOL: **http://search.aol.com/cat.adp?id=169&layer=&from=subcats**
- Chinese Medicine: **http://www.newcenturynutrition.com/**
- drkoop.com®: **http://www.drkoop.com/InteractiveMedicine/IndexC.html**
- Family Village: **http://www.familyvillage.wisc.edu/med_altn.htm**
- Google: **http://directory.google.com/Top/Health/Alternative/**
- Healthnotes: **http://www.healthnotes.com/**
- MedWebPlus: **http://medwebplus.com/subject/Alternative_and_Complementary_Medicine**
- Open Directory Project: **http://dmoz.org/Health/Alternative/**
- HealthGate: **http://www.tnp.com/**
- WebMD®Health: **http://my.webmd.com/drugs_and_herbs**
- WholeHealthMD.com: **http://www.wholehealthmd.com/reflib/0,1529,00.html**
- Yahoo.com: **http://dir.yahoo.com/Health/Alternative_Medicine/**

The following is a specific Web list relating to essential tremor; please note that any particular subject below may indicate either a therapeutic use, or a contraindication (potential danger), and does not reflect an official recommendation:

- **Herbs and Supplements**

  Propranolol
  Source: Healthnotes, Inc.; www.healthnotes.com

General References

A good place to find general background information on CAM is the National Library of Medicine. It has prepared within the MEDLINEplus system an information topic page dedicated to complementary and alternative medicine. To access this page, go to the MEDLINEplus site at **http://www.nlm.nih.gov/medlineplus/alternativemedicine.html**. This Web site provides a general overview of various topics and can lead to a number of general sources.

CHAPTER 3. PATENTS ON ESSENTIAL TREMOR

Overview

Patents can be physical innovations (e.g. chemicals, pharmaceuticals, medical equipment) or processes (e.g. treatments or diagnostic procedures). The United States Patent and Trademark Office defines a patent as a grant of a property right to the inventor, issued by the Patent and Trademark Office.[4] Patents, therefore, are intellectual property. For the United States, the term of a new patent is 20 years from the date when the patent application was filed. If the inventor wishes to receive economic benefits, it is likely that the invention will become commercially available within 20 years of the initial filing. It is important to understand, therefore, that an inventor's patent does not indicate that a product or service is or will be commercially available. The patent implies only that the inventor has "the right to exclude others from making, using, offering for sale, or selling" the invention in the United States. While this relates to U.S. patents, similar rules govern foreign patents.

In this chapter, we show you how to locate information on patents and their inventors. If you find a patent that is particularly interesting to you, contact the inventor or the assignee for further information. **IMPORTANT NOTE:** When following the search strategy described below, you may discover non-medical patents that use the generic term "essential tremor" (or a synonym) in their titles. To accurately reflect the results that you might find while conducting research on essential tremor, we have not necessarily excluded non-medical patents in this bibliography.

Patents on Essential Tremor

By performing a patent search focusing on essential tremor, you can obtain information such as the title of the invention, the names of the inventor(s), the assignee(s) or the company that owns or controls the patent, a short abstract that summarizes the patent, and a few excerpts from the description of the patent. The abstract of a patent tends to be more technical in nature, while the description is often written for the public. Full patent descriptions contain much more information than is presented here (e.g. claims, references, figures, diagrams, etc.). We will tell you how to obtain this information later in the chapter. The following is an

---

[4]Adapted from the United States Patent and Trademark Office:
http://www.uspto.gov/web/offices/pac/doc/general/whatis.htm.

example of the type of information that you can expect to obtain from a patent search on essential tremor:

- **Anticonvulsant derivatives useful in treating essential tremor**

  Inventor(s): Connor; Gregory S. (Tulsa, OK)

  Assignee(s): Ortho-McNeil Pharmaceutical, Inc. (Raritan, NJ)

  Patent Number: 6,214,867

  Date filed: February 15, 2000

  Abstract: Anticonvulsant derivatives useful in treating **essential tremor** are disclosed.

  Excerpt(s): are structurally novel antiepileptic compounds that are highly effective anticonvulsants in animal tests (Maryanoff, B. E, Nortey, S. O., Gardocki, J. F., Shank, R. P. and Dodgson, S. P. J. Med. Chem. 30, 880-887, 1987; Maryanoff, B. E., Costanzo, M. J., Shank, R. P., Schupsky, J. J., Ortegon, M. E., and Vaught J. L. Bioorganic & Medicinal Chemistry Letters 3, 2653-2656, 1993). These compounds are covered by U.S. Pat. No. 4,513,006. One of these compounds 2,3:4,5-bis-O-(1-methylethylidene)-.beta.-D-fructopyranose sulfamate known as topiramate has been demonstrated in clinical trials of human epilepsy to be effective as adjunctive therapy or as monotherapy in treating simple and complex partial seizures and secondarily generalized seizures (E. FAUGHT, B. J. WILDER, R. E. RAMSEY, R. A. REIFE, L. D. KRAMER, G. W. PLEDGER, R. M. KARIM et. al., Epilepsia 36 (S4) 33, 1995; S. K. SACHDEO, R. C. SACHDEO, R. A. REIFE, P. LIM and G. PLEDGER, Epilepsia 36 (S4 33, 1995), and is currently marketed for the treatment of simple and complex partial seizure epilepsy with or without secondary generalized seizures in approximately twenty countries including the United States, and applications for regulatory approval are presently pending in several additional countries throughout the world. Compounds of Formula I were initially found to possess anticonvulsant activity in the traditional maximal electroshock seizure (MES) test in mice (SHANK, R. P., GARDOCKI, J. F., VAUGHT, J. L., DAVIS, C. B., SCHUPSKY, J. J., RAFFA, R. B., DODGSON, S. J., NORTEY, S. O., and MARYANOFF, B. E., Epilepsia 35 450-460, 1994). Subsequent studies revealed that Compounds of Formula I were also highly effective in the MES test in rats. More recently topiramate was found to effectively block seizures in several rodent models of epilepsy (J. NAKAMURA, S. TAMURA, T. KANDA, A. ISHII, K. ISHIHARA, T. SERIKAWA, J. YAMADA, and M. SASA, Eur. J. Pharmacol. 254 83-89, 1994), and in an animal model of kindled epilepsy (A. WAUQUIER and S. ZHOU, Epilepsy Res. 24, 73-77, 1996). The conditions known as familial, essential and senile tremor cannot be distinguished on the basis of physiologic and pharmacologic properties. These are in the class of action tremors that oscillate with a frequency of about 4-8 hz, with variable amplitude. The familial form tends to be inherited as an autosomal trait and can begin in childhood, but typically onset is in adulthood and persists for life. If an inheritance pattern is not evident, the tremor is referred to as an **essential tremor**. **Essential tremor** also known as benign or idiopathic tremor begins early in adult life and persists. If tremor becomes evident in late life, it is known as a senile tremor. For purposes of the present application, the term "essential tremor" as used hereinafter, shall refer to and include familial, essential and senile tremor.

  Web site: http://www.delphion.com/details?pn=US06214867__

- **Hand-held gyroscopic device**

  Inventor(s): Hall; William D. (10850 Stanmore Dr., Potomac, MD 20854)

  Assignee(s): none reported

  Patent Number: 5,058,571

  Date filed: January 22, 1990

  Abstract: A gyroscope is firmly held against the back side of the human hand to reduce or eliminate the effect of naturally occurring tremors such as **essential tremor** or other tremor. The gyroscope is driven by an electric motor energized by batteries. The batteries are mounted near the periphery of the gyroscope to enhance the gyroscopic action. In a modified form of the invention the motor is not mounted on the back side of the hand but is a separate unit to which the gyroscope can be readily coupled and uncoupled.

  Excerpt(s): There is a disease known as "essential tremor" which may involve a tremor in the right hand of a right-handed person or in the left hand of a left-handed person. The effect of the tremor might not impair the person from driving a nail with a hammer but yet might affect delicate work. For example, persons afflicted with **essential tremor** may not be be able to hold a cup of water without spilling it and may not be able to use a spoon to move soup from a bowl to the mouth. In one form of the invention a battery-driven gyroscope is mounted on the back of the hand and rotates at high speed. The batteries are mounted on the rotating part of the gyroscope and add to the gyroscopic action. Another form of the invention employs a gyroscope firmly attached to the back of the hand but without a motor carried by the hand. The motor is mounted on a table where it is readily accessible to the hand held gyroscope. There is a coupling that enables the gyroscope to be driven by the motor. The gyroscope may hold the hand steady long enough to perform a simple task.

  Web site: http://www.delphion.com/details?pn=US05058571__

- **Method and apparatus for treating chronic pain syndromes, tremor, dementia and related disorders and for inducing electroanesthesia using high frequency, high intensity transcutaneous electrical nerve stimulation**

  Inventor(s): Silverstone; Leon M. (La Jolla, CA)

  Assignee(s): Synaptic Corporation (Aurora, CO)

  Patent Number: 6,161,044

  Date filed: November 23, 1998

  Abstract: Provided herein is a non-invasive method of treating, controlling or preventing medical, psychiatric or neurological disorders, using transcutaneous electrical stimulation. The method employs a plurality of stimulation frequency parameters, ranging from a relatively high frequency, for example about 40,000 Hertz, to a relatively low frequency, for example about 250 Hertz, the entire plurality of frequency parameters being administered at each of a plurality of stimulation intensity levels. In particular, the method involves stimulating at a first highest frequency parameter and a first lowest intensity parameter, incrementally decreasing the stimulation frequency parameter a lowest frequency parameter, increasing the frequency parameter to the highest frequency parameter and increasing the intensity parameter to a next highest intensity parameter, and again stimulating through the plurality of frequency parameters from the highest frequency to the lowest frequency. The method described herein is useful in treating, controlling and/or preventing various disease states and disorders, including without limitation, tremor disorders, such as **essential tremor** and Parkinson's disease, dementia disorders, such as Alzheimer's disease and painful degenerative disorders, such as reflex sympathetic dystrophy and fibromyalgia.

Excerpt(s): The present invention relates to improved methods for the non-invasive treatment of various disease conditions using an improved process of transcutaneous electrical stimulation. In particular, provided herein are improved methods of non-invasively treating symptoms of tremor disorders including essential tremors and tremors associated with Parkinson's Disease; symptoms of dementia disorders including cortical dementia, such as is found in Alzheimer's disease and Pick's disease, subcortical dementia, such as is found in Parkinson's disease, Huntington's chorea and supranuclear palsy, and multi-infarct dementia; and symptoms of painful degenerative disorders, such as fibromyalgia and reflex sympathetic dystrophy by using transcutaneous electrical nerve stimulation programs of variable intensity and variable frequency. Also provided are apparatus for performing such methods. Transcutaneous electrical nerve stimulation (TENS) is a well known medical treatment used primarily for symptomatic relief and management of chronic intractable pain and as an adjunctive treatment in the management of post surgical and post traumatic acute pain. TENS involves the application of electrical pulses to the skin of a patient, which pulses are generally of a low frequency and are intended to affect the nervous system in such a way as to suppress the sensation of pain that would indicate acute or chronic injury or otherwise serve as a protective mechanism for the body. Typically, two electrodes are secured to the skin at appropriately selected locations. Mild electrical impulses are then passed into the skin through the electrodes to interact with the nerves lying thereunder. As a symptomatic treatment, TENS has proven to effectively reduce both chronic and acute pain of patients. However, TENS has shown no capacity for curing the causes of pain, rather the electrical energy simply interacts with the nervous system to suppress or relieve pain. The human nervous system essentially serves as a communication system for the body wherein information concerning the state of the body is communicated to the spinal cord (and/or brain) and behavioral instructions are communicated from the brain (and/or spinal cord) to the rest of the body. Thus, there are ascending neural pathways, such as the ascending pain pathways, and descending neural pathways, such as the descending inhibitory pathway (DIP), within the nervous system.

Web site: http://www.delphion.com/details?pn=US06161044__

Patent Applications on Essential Tremor

As of December 2000, U.S. patent applications are open to public viewing.[5] Applications are patent requests which have yet to be granted. (The process to achieve a patent can take several years.) The following patent applications have been filed since December 2000 relating to essential tremor:

---

[5] This has been a common practice outside the United States prior to December 2000.

- **Device driver system for minimizing adverse tremor effects during use of pointing devices**

Inventor(s): Adapathya, Ravi Shankarnarayan; (Durham, NC), Champion, David Frederick; (Durham, NC), Happ, Alan Joseph; (Raleigh, NC), Lawrence, Brad Michael; (Durham, NC), Schultz, Kevin Laverne; (Raleigh, NC)

Correspondence: Ibm Corporation; 2y7/b656; PO Box 12195; Research Triangle Park; NC; 27709; US

Patent Application Number: 20020120217

Date filed: February 26, 2001

Abstract: A system and method for minimizing **essential tremor** effects while utilizing a pointing device on a computer system is disclosed. The system and method comprises obtaining an individual's tremor characteristics and calculating the frequency components of the tremor to obtain digital filter coefficients. The method and system further includes creating a calibration profile comprised of digital filter coefficient that plugs into a pointing device driver; and utilizing the modified device driver to eliminate the effects of the essential tremors. The system and method includes a software tuning algorithm used to obtain an individual's tremor characteristics. A spectral analysis system will calculate the frequency components of the tremor and digital filter coefficients will be saved as a profile. The appropriate filter coefficients will be passed to a device driver via the profile. The modified device driver will filter the pointing device input data based on the filter coefficients and eliminate tremor effects from the on-screen pointer. Because the profile is transferable, if a device driver capable of accepting the profile plug-in were already installed on a computer, the profile could be loaded and used immediately on the computer without the need for re-calibration.

Excerpt(s): The present invention relates generally to computer systems and more particularly to the use of pointing devices in such computer systems. Essential tremor (ET), characterized by rhythmic "back and forth" movement from involuntary musculature contraction, affects as many as 1 in 20 people over 40 and 1 in 5 people over 65. With the exception of stroke, **essential tremor** is more common than any other neurological disease, affecting over 5 million Americans. It is very difficult for people with ET to effectively use a handheld computer pointing device, such as a mouse, due to continuous hand displacement caused by tremor. Tracking tasks and tasks where the individual must click on a small target (e.g., the "close window" button in a graphical user interface) are especially difficult. Accordingly, what is needed is a system and method for responding to essential tremors when using a pointing device that is simple, easy to implement and is acceptable to many different individuals. The present invention addresses such a need.

Web site: http://appft1.uspto.gov/netahtml/PTO/search-bool.html

- **Method for treating essential tremor with botulinum toxin type B**

Inventor(s): Aoki, K. Roger; (Laguna Hill, CA), Carlson, Steven R.; (Laguna Niguel, CA), Grayston, Michael W.; (Irvine, CA), Leon, Judith M.; (Laguna Niguel, CA)

Correspondence: Stephen Donovan; Allergan, INC.; 2525 Dupont Drive; Irvine; CA; 92612; US

Patent Application Number: 20010041181

Date filed: June 15, 2001

Abstract: A method and composition for treating a patient suffering from a disease, disorder or condition and associated pain include the administration to the patient of a therapeutically effective amount of a neurotoxin selected from a group consisting of Botulinum toxin types A, B, C, D, E, F and G.

Excerpt(s): The present invention provides novel methods for treating various disorders and conditions, with Botulinum toxins. Importantly, the present invention provides methods useful in relieving pain related to muscle activity or contracture and therefore is of advantage in the treatment of, for example, muscle spasm such as Temporomandibular Joint Disease, low back pain, myofascial pain, pain related to spasticity and dystonia, as well as sports injuries, and pain related to contractures in arthritis. Heretofore, Botulinum toxins, in particular Botulinum toxin type A, has been used in the treatment of a number of neuromuscular disorders and conditions involving muscular spasm; for example, strabismus, blepharospasm, spasmodic torticollis (cervical dystonia), oromandibular dystonia and spasmodic dysphonia (laryngeal dystonia). The toxin binds rapidly and strongly to presynaptic cholinergic nerve terminals and inhibits the exocytosis of acetylcholine by decreasing the frequency of acetylcholine release. This results in local paralysis and hence relaxation of the muscle afflicted by spasm. For one example of treating neuromuscular disorders, see U.S. Pat. No. 5,053,005 to Borodic, which suggests treating curvature of the juvenile spine, i.e., scoliosis, with an acetylcholine release inhibitor, preferably Botulinum toxin A.

Web site: http://appft1.uspto.gov/netahtml/PTO/search-bool.html

- **Methods for treating essential tremor**

  Inventor(s): Gliner, Bradford Evan; (Sammamish, WA), Wyler, Allen; (Seattle, WA)

  Correspondence: Perkins Coie Llp; Patent-Sea; P.O. Box 1247; Seattle; WA; 98111-1247; US

  Patent Application Number: 20040111129

  Date filed: July 17, 2003

  Abstract: Methods for treating **essential tremor** are disclosed. A method in accordance with one embodiment of the invention includes directing a patient to perform a muscle action, for example, a postural or kinetic muscle action. The method can further include directing information to be collected, with the information corresponding to a level of neural activity in the patient's brain while the patient performs the muscle action. The **essential tremor** motion of the patient can then be at least reduced by applying an electrical stimulation at least proximate to a stimulation site, with the location of the stimulation site being based at least in part on the collected information. The information can include visual images, such as are generated by MRI, fMRI, or CT techniques, or the information can be non-visual. In particular embodiments, the location of the stimulation site can be determined by comparing two pieces of information, for example, neural activities before and after drug intake, or neural activities at the left and right hemispheres of the brain.

  Excerpt(s): The present application claims priority to pending U.S. Provisional Application 60/432,073, entitled "System and Method for Treating Parkinson's Disease and other Movement Disorders," filed Dec. 9, 2002. The present invention is directed toward systems and methods for treating **essential tremor,** associated with abnormal neural activity in the brain. A wide variety of mental and physical processes are controlled or influenced by neural activity in particular regions of the brain. For example, various physical or cognitive functions are directed or affected by neural activity within the sensory or motor cortices. Across most individuals, particular areas of the brain appear to have distinct functions. In the majority of people, for example, the areas of the occipital lobes relate to vision; the regions of the left interior frontal lobes relate to language; portions of the cerebral cortex appear to be consistently involved with conscious awareness, memory, and intellect; and particular regions of the cerebral cortex as well as the basal ganglia, the thalamus, and the motor cortex cooperatively interact to facilitate motor function control.

Web site: http://appft1.uspto.gov/netahtml/PTO/search-bool.html

Keeping Current

In order to stay informed about patents and patent applications dealing with essential tremor, you can access the U.S. Patent Office archive via the Internet at the following Web address: **http://www.uspto.gov/patft/index.html**. You will see two broad options: (1) Issued Patent, and (2) Published Applications. To see a list of issued patents, perform the following steps: Under "Issued Patents," click "Quick Search." Then, type "essential tremor" (or synonyms) into the "Term 1" box. After clicking on the search button, scroll down to see the various patents which have been granted to date on essential tremor.

You can also use this procedure to view pending patent applications concerning essential tremor. Simply go back to **http://www.uspto.gov/patft/index.html**. Select "Quick Search" under "Published Applications." Then proceed with the steps listed above.

CHAPTER 4. BOOKS ON ESSENTIAL TREMOR

Overview

This chapter provides bibliographic book references relating to essential tremor. In addition to online booksellers such as **www.amazon.com** and **www.bn.com**, excellent sources for book titles on essential tremor include the Combined Health Information Database and the National Library of Medicine. Your local medical library also may have these titles available for loan.

Book Summaries: Federal Agencies

The Combined Health Information Database collects various book abstracts from a variety of healthcare institutions and federal agencies. To access these summaries, go directly to the following hyperlink: **http://chid.nih.gov/detail/detail.html**. You will need to use the "Detailed Search" option. To find book summaries, use the drop boxes at the bottom of the search page where "You may refine your search by." Select the dates and language you prefer. For the format option, select "Monograph/Book." Now type "essential tremor" (or synonyms) into the "For these words:" box. You should check back periodically with this database which is updated every three months. The following is a typical result when searching for books on essential tremor:

- **Handbook of Tremor Disorders**

  Source: New York, NY: Marcel Dekker, Inc. 1995. 576 p.

  Contact: Available from Marcel Dekker, Inc., Cimarron Road, P.O. Box 5005, Monticello, NY 12701. (845) 796-1919. Toll-free: (800) 228- 1160. Fax: (845) 796-1772. E-mail: custserv@dekker.com. Web site: www.dekker.com. ISBN: 0-8247-8859-1. PRICE: $235.00 plus shipping, tax, and handling. Available in hardcover.

  Summary: Tremors are a common phenomenon presented to physicians and can be diagnosed as a condition or a symptom of a disorder of the nervous system. Written by clinical and research scientists, this reference examines the mechanisms of tremor, assessment procedures, diagnosis, and treatment. Specific topics include definitions and classifications, causes, pharmacological management, challenges in measurement, differential diagnoses, normal tremors in the elderly, and surgical options. **Essential**

tremor, Parkinsonian tremor, cerebellar tremors, orthostatis tremor, dystonia, midbrain tremor, and tremor in AIDS are addressed.

CHAPTER 5. PERIODICALS AND NEWS ON ESSENTIAL TREMOR

Overview

In this chapter, we suggest a number of news sources and present various periodicals that cover essential tremor.

News Services and Press Releases

One of the simplest ways of tracking press releases on essential tremor is to search the news wires. In the following sample of sources, we will briefly describe how to access each service. These services only post recent news intended for public viewing.

PR Newswire

To access the PR Newswire archive, simply go to **http://www.prnewswire.com/**. Select your country. Type "essential tremor" (or synonyms) into the search box. You will automatically receive information on relevant news releases posted within the last 30 days. The search results are shown by order of relevance.

Reuters Health

The Reuters' Medical News and Health eLine databases can be very useful in exploring news archives relating to essential tremor. While some of the listed articles are free to view, others are available for purchase for a nominal fee. To access this archive, go to **http://www.reutershealth.com/en/index.html** and search by "essential tremor" (or synonyms). The following was recently listed in this archive for essential tremor:

- **Gene Locus For Essential Tremor Located**
  Source: Reuters Medical News
  Date: November 10, 1997

- **Location Of Gene For Familial Essential Tremor Identified**
  Source: Reuters Medical News
  Date: August 27, 1997

The NIH

Within MEDLINEplus, the NIH has made an agreement with the New York Times Syndicate, the AP News Service, and Reuters to deliver news that can be browsed by the public. Search news releases at **http://www.nlm.nih.gov/medlineplus/alphanews_a.html**. MEDLINEplus allows you to browse across an alphabetical index. Or you can search by date at the following Web page: **http://www.nlm.nih.gov/medlineplus/newsbydate.html**. Often, news items are indexed by MEDLINEplus within its search engine.

Business Wire

Business Wire is similar to PR Newswire. To access this archive, simply go to **http://www.businesswire.com/**. You can scan the news by industry category or company name.

Market Wire

Market Wire is more focused on technology than the other wires. To browse the latest press releases by topic, such as alternative medicine, biotechnology, fitness, healthcare, legal, nutrition, and pharmaceuticals, access Market Wire's Medical/Health channel at **http://www.marketwire.com/mw/release_index?channel=MedicalHealth**. Or simply go to Market Wire's home page at **http://www.marketwire.com/mw/home**, type "essential tremor" (or synonyms) into the search box, and click on "Search News." As this service is technology oriented, you may wish to use it when searching for press releases covering diagnostic procedures or tests.

Search Engines

Medical news is also available in the news sections of commercial Internet search engines. See the health news page at Yahoo (**http://dir.yahoo.com/Health/News_and_Media/**), or you can use this Web site's general news search page at **http://news.yahoo.com/**. Type in "essential tremor" (or synonyms). If you know the name of a company that is relevant to essential tremor, you can go to any stock trading Web site (such as **http://www.etrade.com/**) and search for the company name there. News items across various news sources are reported on indicated hyperlinks. Google offers a similar service at **http://news.google.com/**.

BBC

Covering news from a more European perspective, the British Broadcasting Corporation (BBC) allows the public free access to their news archive located at **http://www.bbc.co.uk/**. Search by "essential tremor" (or synonyms).

Academic Periodicals covering Essential Tremor

Numerous periodicals are currently indexed within the National Library of Medicine's PubMed database that are known to publish articles relating to essential tremor. In addition to these sources, you can search for articles covering essential tremor that have been published by any of the periodicals listed in previous chapters. To find the latest studies published, go to **http://www.ncbi.nlm.nih.gov/pubmed**, type the name of the periodical into the search box, and click "Go."

If you want complete details about the historical contents of a journal, you can also visit the following Web site: **http://www.ncbi.nlm.nih.gov/entrez/jrbrowser.cgi**. Here, type in the name of the journal or its abbreviation, and you will receive an index of published articles. At **http://locatorplus.gov/**, you can retrieve more indexing information on medical periodicals (e.g. the name of the publisher). Select the button "Search LOCATORplus." Then type in the name of the journal and select the advanced search option "Journal Title Search."

CHAPTER 6. RESEARCHING MEDICATIONS

Overview

While a number of hard copy or CD-ROM resources are available for researching medications, a more flexible method is to use Internet-based databases. Broadly speaking, there are two sources of information on approved medications: public sources and private sources. We will emphasize free-to-use public sources.

U.S. Pharmacopeia

Because of historical investments by various organizations and the emergence of the Internet, it has become rather simple to learn about the medications recommended for essential tremor. One such source is the United States Pharmacopeia. In 1820, eleven physicians met in Washington, D.C. to establish the first compendium of standard drugs for the United States. They called this compendium the U.S. Pharmacopeia (USP). Today, the USP is a non-profit organization consisting of 800 volunteer scientists, eleven elected officials, and 400 representatives of state associations and colleges of medicine and pharmacy. The USP is located in Rockville, Maryland, and its home page is located at **http://www.usp.org/**. The USP currently provides standards for over 3,700 medications. The resulting USP DI® Advice for the Patient® can be accessed through the National Library of Medicine of the National Institutes of Health. The database is partially derived from lists of federally approved medications in the Food and Drug Administration's (FDA) Drug Approvals database, located at **http://www.fda.gov/cder/da/da.htm**.

While the FDA database is rather large and difficult to navigate, the Phamacopeia is both user-friendly and free to use. It covers more than 9,000 prescription and over-the-counter medications. To access this database, simply type the following hyperlink into your Web browser: **http://www.nlm.nih.gov/medlineplus/druginformation.html**. To view examples of a given medication (brand names, category, description, preparation, proper use, precautions, side effects, etc.), simply follow the hyperlinks indicated within the United States Pharmacopeia (USP).

Below, we have compiled a list of medications associated with essential tremor. If you would like more information on a particular medication, the provided hyperlinks will direct you to ample documentation (e.g. typical dosage, side effects, drug-interaction risks, etc.).

The following drugs have been mentioned in the Pharmacopeia and other sources as being potentially applicable to essential tremor:

Caffeine

- **Systemic - U.S. Brands:** Cafcit; Caffedrine Caplets; Dexitac Stay Alert Stimulant; Enerjets; Keep Alert; Maximum Strength SnapBack Stimulant Powders; NoDoz Maximum Strength Caplets; Pep-Back; Quick Pep; Ultra Pep-Back; Vivarin
  http://www.nlm.nih.gov/medlineplus/druginfo/uspdi/202105.html

Primidone

- **Systemic - U.S. Brands:** Myidone; Mysoline
  http://www.nlm.nih.gov/medlineplus/druginfo/uspdi/202479.html

Commercial Databases

In addition to the medications listed in the USP above, a number of commercial sites are available by subscription to physicians and their institutions. Or, you may be able to access these sources from your local medical library.

Mosby's Drug Consult™

Mosby's Drug Consult™ database (also available on CD-ROM and book format) covers 45,000 drug products including generics and international brands. It provides prescribing information, drug interactions, and patient information. Subscription information is available at the following hyperlink: **http://www.mosbysdrugconsult.com/**.

PDR*health*

The PDR*health* database is a free-to-use, drug information search engine that has been written for the public in layman's terms. It contains FDA-approved drug information adapted from the Physicians' Desk Reference (PDR) database. PDR*health* can be searched by brand name, generic name, or indication. It features multiple drug interactions reports. Search PDR*health* at **http://www.pdrhealth.com/drug_info/index.html**.

Other Web Sites

Drugs.com (**www.drugs.com**) reproduces the information in the Pharmacopeia as well as commercial information. You may also want to consider the Web site of the Medical Letter, Inc. (**http://www.medletter.com/**) which allows users to download articles on various drugs and therapeutics for a nominal fee.

If you have any questions about a medical treatment, the FDA may have an office near you. Look for their number in the blue pages of the phone book. You can also contact the FDA through its toll-free number, 1-888-INFO-FDA (1-888-463-6332), or on the World Wide Web at **www.fda.gov**.

APPENDICES

APPENDIX A. PHYSICIAN RESOURCES

Overview

In this chapter, we focus on databases and Internet-based guidelines and information resources created or written for a professional audience.

NIH Guidelines

Commonly referred to as "clinical" or "professional" guidelines, the National Institutes of Health publish physician guidelines for the most common diseases. Publications are available at the following by relevant Institute[6]:

- Office of the Director (OD); guidelines consolidated across agencies available at **http://www.nih.gov/health/consumer/conkey.htm**

- National Institute of General Medical Sciences (NIGMS); fact sheets available at **http://www.nigms.nih.gov/news/facts/**

- National Library of Medicine (NLM); extensive encyclopedia (A.D.A.M., Inc.) with guidelines: **http://www.nlm.nih.gov/medlineplus/healthtopics.html**

- National Cancer Institute (NCI); guidelines available at **http://www.cancer.gov/cancerinfo/list.aspx?viewid=5f35036e-5497-4d86-8c2c-714a9f7c8d25**

- National Eye Institute (NEI); guidelines available at **http://www.nei.nih.gov/order/index.htm**

- National Heart, Lung, and Blood Institute (NHLBI); guidelines available at **http://www.nhlbi.nih.gov/guidelines/index.htm**

- National Human Genome Research Institute (NHGRI); research available at **http://www.genome.gov/page.cfm?pageID=10000375**

- National Institute on Aging (NIA); guidelines available at **http://www.nia.nih.gov/health/**

---

[6] These publications are typically written by one or more of the various NIH Institutes.

- National Institute on Alcohol Abuse and Alcoholism (NIAAA); guidelines available at http://www.niaaa.nih.gov/publications/publications.htm

- National Institute of Allergy and Infectious Diseases (NIAID); guidelines available at http://www.niaid.nih.gov/publications/

- National Institute of Arthritis and Musculoskeletal and Skin Diseases (NIAMS); fact sheets and guidelines available at http://www.niams.nih.gov/hi/index.htm

- National Institute of Child Health and Human Development (NICHD); guidelines available at http://www.nichd.nih.gov/publications/pubskey.cfm

- National Institute on Deafness and Other Communication Disorders (NIDCD); fact sheets and guidelines at http://www.nidcd.nih.gov/health/

- National Institute of Dental and Craniofacial Research (NIDCR); guidelines available at http://www.nidr.nih.gov/health/

- National Institute of Diabetes and Digestive and Kidney Diseases (NIDDK); guidelines available at http://www.niddk.nih.gov/health/health.htm

- National Institute on Drug Abuse (NIDA); guidelines available at http://www.nida.nih.gov/DrugAbuse.html

- National Institute of Environmental Health Sciences (NIEHS); environmental health information available at http://www.niehs.nih.gov/external/facts.htm

- National Institute of Mental Health (NIMH); guidelines available at http://www.nimh.nih.gov/practitioners/index.cfm

- National Institute of Neurological Disorders and Stroke (NINDS); neurological disorder information pages available at http://www.ninds.nih.gov/health_and_medical/disorder_index.htm

- National Institute of Nursing Research (NINR); publications on selected illnesses at http://www.nih.gov/ninr/news-info/publications.html

- National Institute of Biomedical Imaging and Bioengineering; general information at http://grants.nih.gov/grants/becon/becon_info.htm

- Center for Information Technology (CIT); referrals to other agencies based on keyword searches available at http://kb.nih.gov/www_query_main.asp

- National Center for Complementary and Alternative Medicine (NCCAM); health information available at http://nccam.nih.gov/health/

- National Center for Research Resources (NCRR); various information directories available at http://www.ncrr.nih.gov/publications.asp

- Office of Rare Diseases; various fact sheets available at http://rarediseases.info.nih.gov/html/resources/rep_pubs.html

- Centers for Disease Control and Prevention; various fact sheets on infectious diseases available at http://www.cdc.gov/publications.htm

NIH Databases

In addition to the various Institutes of Health that publish professional guidelines, the NIH has designed a number of databases for professionals.[7] Physician-oriented resources provide a wide variety of information related to the biomedical and health sciences, both past and present. The format of these resources varies. Searchable databases, bibliographic citations, full-text articles (when available), archival collections, and images are all available. The following are referenced by the National Library of Medicine:[8]

- **Bioethics:** Access to published literature on the ethical, legal, and public policy issues surrounding healthcare and biomedical research. This information is provided in conjunction with the Kennedy Institute of Ethics located at Georgetown University, Washington, D.C.: **http://www.nlm.nih.gov/databases/databases_bioethics.html**

- **HIV/AIDS Resources:** Describes various links and databases dedicated to HIV/AIDS research: **http://www.nlm.nih.gov/pubs/factsheets/aidsinfs.html**

- **NLM Online Exhibitions:** Describes "Exhibitions in the History of Medicine": **http://www.nlm.nih.gov/exhibition/exhibition.html**. Additional resources for historical scholarship in medicine: **http://www.nlm.nih.gov/hmd/hmd.html**

- **Biotechnology Information:** Access to public databases. The National Center for Biotechnology Information conducts research in computational biology, develops software tools for analyzing genome data, and disseminates biomedical information for the better understanding of molecular processes affecting human health and disease: **http://www.ncbi.nlm.nih.gov/**

- **Population Information:** The National Library of Medicine provides access to worldwide coverage of population, family planning, and related health issues, including family planning technology and programs, fertility, and population law and policy: **http://www.nlm.nih.gov/databases/databases_population.html**

- **Cancer Information:** Access to cancer-oriented databases: **http://www.nlm.nih.gov/databases/databases_cancer.html**

- **Profiles in Science:** Offering the archival collections of prominent twentieth-century biomedical scientists to the public through modern digital technology: **http://www.profiles.nlm.nih.gov/**

- **Chemical Information:** Provides links to various chemical databases and references: **http://sis.nlm.nih.gov/Chem/ChemMain.html**

- **Clinical Alerts:** Reports the release of findings from the NIH-funded clinical trials where such release could significantly affect morbidity and mortality: **http://www.nlm.nih.gov/databases/alerts/clinical_alerts.html**

- **Space Life Sciences:** Provides links and information to space-based research (including NASA): **http://www.nlm.nih.gov/databases/databases_space.html**

- **MEDLINE:** Bibliographic database covering the fields of medicine, nursing, dentistry, veterinary medicine, the healthcare system, and the pre-clinical sciences: **http://www.nlm.nih.gov/databases/databases_medline.html**

---

[7] Remember, for the general public, the National Library of Medicine recommends the databases referenced in MEDLINE*plus* (**http://medlineplus.gov/** or **http://www.nlm.nih.gov/medlineplus/databases.html**).

[8] See **http://www.nlm.nih.gov/databases/databases.html**.

- **Toxicology and Environmental Health Information (TOXNET):** Databases covering toxicology and environmental health: **http://sis.nlm.nih.gov/Tox/ToxMain.html**

- **Visible Human Interface:** Anatomically detailed, three-dimensional representations of normal male and female human bodies: **http://www.nlm.nih.gov/research/visible/visible_human.html**

The NLM Gateway[9]

The NLM (National Library of Medicine) Gateway is a Web-based system that lets users search simultaneously in multiple retrieval systems at the U.S. National Library of Medicine (NLM). It allows users of NLM services to initiate searches from one Web interface, providing one-stop searching for many of NLM's information resources or databases.[10] To use the NLM Gateway, simply go to the search site at **http://gateway.nlm.nih.gov/gw/Cmd**. Type "essential tremor" (or synonyms) into the search box and click "Search." The results will be presented in a tabular form, indicating the number of references in each database category.

Results Summary

Category	Items Found
Journal Articles	1133
Books / Periodicals / Audio Visual	8
Consumer Health	313
Meeting Abstracts	2
Other Collections	32
Total	1488

HSTAT[11]

HSTAT is a free, Web-based resource that provides access to full-text documents used in healthcare decision-making.[12] These documents include clinical practice guidelines, quick-reference guides for clinicians, consumer health brochures, evidence reports and technology assessments from the Agency for Healthcare Research and Quality (AHRQ), as well as AHRQ's Put Prevention Into Practice.[13] Simply search by "essential tremor" (or synonyms) at the following Web site: **http://text.nlm.nih.gov**.

---

[9] Adapted from NLM: **http://gateway.nlm.nih.gov/gw/Cmd?Overview.x**.

[10] The NLM Gateway is currently being developed by the Lister Hill National Center for Biomedical Communications (LHNCBC) at the National Library of Medicine (NLM) of the National Institutes of Health (NIH).

[11] Adapted from HSTAT: **http://www.nlm.nih.gov/pubs/factsheets/hstat.html**.

[12] The HSTAT URL is **http://hstat.nlm.nih.gov/**.

[13] Other important documents in HSTAT include: the National Institutes of Health (NIH) Consensus Conference Reports and Technology Assessment Reports; the HIV/AIDS Treatment Information Service (ATIS) resource documents; the Substance Abuse and Mental Health Services Administration's Center for Substance Abuse Treatment (SAMHSA/CSAT) Treatment Improvement Protocols (TIP) and Center for Substance Abuse Prevention (SAMHSA/CSAP) Prevention Enhancement Protocols System (PEPS); the Public Health Service (PHS) Preventive Services Task Force's *Guide to Clinical Preventive Services*; the independent, nonfederal Task Force on Community Services' *Guide to Community Preventive Services*; and the Health Technology Advisory Committee (HTAC) of the Minnesota Health Care Commission (MHCC) health technology evaluations.

Coffee Break: Tutorials for Biologists[14]

Coffee Break is a general healthcare site that takes a scientific view of the news and covers recent breakthroughs in biology that may one day assist physicians in developing treatments. Here you will find a collection of short reports on recent biological discoveries. Each report incorporates interactive tutorials that demonstrate how bioinformatics tools are used as a part of the research process. Currently, all Coffee Breaks are written by NCBI staff.[15] Each report is about 400 words and is usually based on a discovery reported in one or more articles from recently published, peer-reviewed literature.[16] This site has new articles every few weeks, so it can be considered an online magazine of sorts. It is intended for general background information. You can access the Coffee Break Web site at the following hyperlink: **http://www.ncbi.nlm.nih.gov/Coffeebreak/**.

Other Commercial Databases

In addition to resources maintained by official agencies, other databases exist that are commercial ventures addressing medical professionals. Here are some examples that may interest you:

- **CliniWeb International:** Index and table of contents to selected clinical information on the Internet; see **http://www.ohsu.edu/cliniweb/**.

- **Medical World Search:** Searches full text from thousands of selected medical sites on the Internet; see **http://www.mwsearch.com/**.

---

[14] Adapted from **http://www.ncbi.nlm.nih.gov/Coffeebreak/Archive/FAQ.html**.

[15] The figure that accompanies each article is frequently supplied by an expert external to NCBI, in which case the source of the figure is cited. The result is an interactive tutorial that tells a biological story.

[16] After a brief introduction that sets the work described into a broader context, the report focuses on how a molecular understanding can provide explanations of observed biology and lead to therapies for diseases. Each vignette is accompanied by a figure and hypertext links that lead to a series of pages that interactively show how NCBI tools and resources are used in the research process.

Appendix B. Patient Resources

Overview

Official agencies, as well as federally funded institutions supported by national grants, frequently publish a variety of guidelines written with the patient in mind. These are typically called "Fact Sheets" or "Guidelines." They can take the form of a brochure, information kit, pamphlet, or flyer. Often they are only a few pages in length. Since new guidelines on essential tremor can appear at any moment and be published by a number of sources, the best approach to finding guidelines is to systematically scan the Internet-based services that post them.

Patient Guideline Sources

The remainder of this chapter directs you to sources which either publish or can help you find additional guidelines on topics related to essential tremor. Due to space limitations, these sources are listed in a concise manner. Do not hesitate to consult the following sources by either using the Internet hyperlink provided, or, in cases where the contact information is provided, contacting the publisher or author directly.

The National Institutes of Health

The NIH gateway to patients is located at **http://health.nih.gov/**. From this site, you can search across various sources and institutes, a number of which are summarized below.

Topic Pages: MEDLINEplus

The National Library of Medicine has created a vast and patient-oriented healthcare information portal called MEDLINEplus. Within this Internet-based system are "health topic pages" which list links to available materials relevant to essential tremor. To access this system, log on to **http://www.nlm.nih.gov/medlineplus/healthtopics.html**. From there you can either search using the alphabetical index or browse by broad topic areas. Recently, MEDLINEplus listed the following when searched for "essential tremor":

Movement Disorders
http://www.nlm.nih.gov/medlineplus/movementdisorders.html

Multiple Sclerosis
http://www.nlm.nih.gov/medlineplus/multiplesclerosis.html

Parkinson's Disease
http://www.nlm.nih.gov/medlineplus/parkinsonsdisease.html

Tremor
http://www.nlm.nih.gov/medlineplus/tremor.html

You may also choose to use the search utility provided by MEDLINEplus at the following Web address: **http://www.nlm.nih.gov/medlineplus/**. Simply type a keyword into the search box and click "Search." This utility is similar to the NIH search utility, with the exception that it only includes materials that are linked within the MEDLINEplus system (mostly patient-oriented information). It also has the disadvantage of generating unstructured results. We recommend, therefore, that you use this method only if you have a very targeted search.

The Combined Health Information Database (CHID)

CHID Online is a reference tool that maintains a database directory of thousands of journal articles and patient education guidelines on essential tremor. CHID offers summaries that describe the guidelines available, including contact information and pricing. CHID's general Web site is **http://chid.nih.gov/**. To search this database, go to **http://chid.nih.gov/detail/detail.html**. In particular, you can use the advanced search options to look up pamphlets, reports, brochures, and information kits. The following was recently posted in this archive:

- **Parkinson's Disease**

  Source: Danbury, CT: National Organization for Rare Disorders, Inc. 2001. 12 p.

  Contact: National Organization for Rare Disorders, Inc. (NORD). P. O. Box 1968, Danbury, CT 06813-1968. (203) 744-0100; (800) 999-6673; TDD (203) 797-9590. E-mail: orphan@rarediseases.org. Website: www.rarediseases.org. PRICE: Free for 1st copy, $7.50 per each additional copy.

  Summary: This fact sheet from the National Organization for Rare Disorders presents comprehensive information on Parkinson's Disease, a slowly progressive neurologic condition characterized by involuntary trembling, muscular stiffness or inflexibility, slowness of movement, and difficulty moving. The general discussion covers symptoms, causes, the affected population, standard and investigational therapies, as well as related disorders such as juvenile parkinsonism of Hunt, Parkinsonism dementia complex, drug-induced parkinsonism, Benign **Essential Tremor,** Hallervorden-Spatz Disease, Olivopontocerebellar Atrophy, Progressive Supranuclear Palsy (PSP), and Shy-Drager Syndrome. Additional contacts and resources are listed. 35 references.

The NIH Search Utility

The NIH search utility allows you to search for documents on over 100 selected Web sites that comprise the NIH-WEB-SPACE. Each of these servers is "crawled" and indexed on an ongoing basis. Your search will produce a list of various documents, all of which will relate in some way to essential tremor. The drawbacks of this approach are that the information is not organized by theme and that the references are often a mix of information for professionals and patients. Nevertheless, a large number of the listed Web sites provide useful background information. We can only recommend this route, therefore, for relatively rare or specific disorders, or when using highly targeted searches. To use the NIH search utility, visit the following Web page: **http://search.nih.gov/index.html**.

PEDBASE

Similar to NORD, PEDBASE covers relatively rare disorders, limited mainly to pediatric conditions. PEDBASE was designed by Dr. Alan Gandy. To access the database, which is more oriented to researchers than patients, you can view the current list of health topics covered at the following Web site: **http://www.icondata.com/health/pedbase/pedlynx.htm**.

Additional Web Sources

A number of Web sites are available to the public that often link to government sites. These can also point you in the direction of essential information. The following is a representative sample:

- AOL: **http://search.aol.com/cat.adp?id=168&layer=&from=subcats**
- Family Village: **http://www.familyvillage.wisc.edu/specific.htm**
- Google: **http://directory.google.com/Top/Health/Conditions_and_Diseases/**
- Med Help International: **http://www.medhelp.org/HealthTopics/A.html**
- Open Directory Project: **http://dmoz.org/Health/Conditions_and_Diseases/**
- Yahoo.com: **http://dir.yahoo.com/Health/Diseases_and_Conditions/**
- WebMD®Health: **http://my.webmd.com/health_topics**

Associations and Essential Tremor

The following is a list of associations that provide information on and resources relating to essential tremor:

- **International Essential Tremor Foundation**

  Telephone: (913) 341-3880 Toll-free: (888) 387-3667

  Fax: (913) 341-1296

  Email: Staff@essentialtremor.org

  Web Site: www.essentialtremors.org

  Background: The International Tremor Foundation (ITF) is a source of information on **essential tremor** for patients, families, and physicians worldwide. The ITF was created to provide information, services, and support to individuals and families affected by **essential tremor** (ET). The organization encourages and promotes research in an effort to determine the cause(s), treatment(s), and ultimately the cure(s) for ET. The ITF is the only worldwide organization dedicated to meeting the needs of those whose daily lives are challenged by ET. The ITF maintains an extensive international referrals service composed of knowledgeable movement disorder neurologists who assist patients and families in receiving correct diagnoses and treatment. These referrals are available upon request.

Relevant area(s) of interest: Essential Tremor

Finding Associations

There are several Internet directories that provide lists of medical associations with information on or resources relating to essential tremor. By consulting all of associations listed in this chapter, you will have nearly exhausted all sources for patient associations concerned with essential tremor.

The National Health Information Center (NHIC)

The National Health Information Center (NHIC) offers a free referral service to help people find organizations that provide information about essential tremor. For more information, see the NHIC's Web site at **http://www.health.gov/NHIC/** or contact an information specialist by calling 1-800-336-4797.

Directory of Health Organizations

The Directory of Health Organizations, provided by the National Library of Medicine Specialized Information Services, is a comprehensive source of information on associations. The Directory of Health Organizations database can be accessed via the Internet at **http://www.sis.nlm.nih.gov/Dir/DirMain.html**. It is composed of two parts: DIRLINE and Health Hotlines.

The DIRLINE database comprises some 10,000 records of organizations, research centers, and government institutes and associations that primarily focus on health and biomedicine. To access DIRLINE directly, go to the following Web site: **http://dirline.nlm.nih.gov/**. Simply type in "essential tremor" (or a synonym), and you will receive information on all relevant organizations listed in the database.

Health Hotlines directs you to toll-free numbers to over 300 organizations. You can access this database directly at **http://www.sis.nlm.nih.gov/hotlines/**. On this page, you are given the option to search by keyword or by browsing the subject list. When you have received your search results, click on the name of the organization for its description and contact information.

The Combined Health Information Database

Another comprehensive source of information on healthcare associations is the Combined Health Information Database. Using the "Detailed Search" option, you will need to limit your search to "Organizations" and "essential tremor". Type the following hyperlink into your Web browser: **http://chid.nih.gov/detail/detail.html**. To find associations, use the drop boxes at the bottom of the search page where "You may refine your search by." For publication date, select "All Years." Then, select your preferred language and the format option "Organization Resource Sheet." Type "essential tremor" (or synonyms) into the "For these words:" box. You should check back periodically with this database since it is updated every three months.

The National Organization for Rare Disorders, Inc.

The National Organization for Rare Disorders, Inc. has prepared a Web site that provides, at no charge, lists of associations organized by health topic. You can access this database at the following Web site: **http://www.rarediseases.org/search/orgsearch.html**. Type "essential tremor" (or a synonym) into the search box, and click "Submit Query."

APPENDIX C. FINDING MEDICAL LIBRARIES

Overview

In this Appendix, we show you how to quickly find a medical library in your area.

Preparation

Your local public library and medical libraries have interlibrary loan programs with the National Library of Medicine (NLM), one of the largest medical collections in the world. According to the NLM, most of the literature in the general and historical collections of the National Library of Medicine is available on interlibrary loan to any library. If you would like to access NLM medical literature, then visit a library in your area that can request the publications for you.[17]

Finding a Local Medical Library

The quickest method to locate medical libraries is to use the Internet-based directory published by the National Network of Libraries of Medicine (NN/LM). This network includes 4626 members and affiliates that provide many services to librarians, health professionals, and the public. To find a library in your area, simply visit **http://nnlm.gov/members/adv.html** or call 1-800-338-7657.

Medical Libraries in the U.S. and Canada

In addition to the NN/LM, the National Library of Medicine (NLM) lists a number of libraries with reference facilities that are open to the public. The following is the NLM's list and includes hyperlinks to each library's Web site. These Web pages can provide information on hours of operation and other restrictions. The list below is a small sample of

---

[17] Adapted from the NLM: **http://www.nlm.nih.gov/psd/cas/interlibrary.html**.

libraries recommended by the National Library of Medicine (sorted alphabetically by name of the U.S. state or Canadian province where the library is located)[18]:

- **Alabama:** Health InfoNet of Jefferson County (Jefferson County Library Cooperative, Lister Hill Library of the Health Sciences), **http://www.uab.edu/infonet/**

- **Alabama:** Richard M. Scrushy Library (American Sports Medicine Institute)

- **Arizona:** Samaritan Regional Medical Center: The Learning Center (Samaritan Health System, Phoenix, Arizona), **http://www.samaritan.edu/library/bannerlibs.htm**

- **California:** Kris Kelly Health Information Center (St. Joseph Health System, Humboldt), **http://www.humboldt1.com/~kkhic/index.html**

- **California:** Community Health Library of Los Gatos, **http://www.healthlib.org/orgresources.html**

- **California:** Consumer Health Program and Services (CHIPS) (County of Los Angeles Public Library, Los Angeles County Harbor-UCLA Medical Center Library) - Carson, CA, **http://www.colapublib.org/services/chips.html**

- **California:** Gateway Health Library (Sutter Gould Medical Foundation)

- **California:** Health Library (Stanford University Medical Center), **http://www-med.stanford.edu/healthlibrary/**

- **California:** Patient Education Resource Center - Health Information and Resources (University of California, San Francisco), **http://sfghdean.ucsf.edu/barnett/PERC/default.asp**

- **California:** Redwood Health Library (Petaluma Health Care District), **http://www.phcd.org/rdwdlib.html**

- **California:** Los Gatos PlaneTree Health Library, **http://planetreesanjose.org/**

- **California:** Sutter Resource Library (Sutter Hospitals Foundation, Sacramento), **http://suttermedicalcenter.org/library/**

- **California:** Health Sciences Libraries (University of California, Davis), **http://www.lib.ucdavis.edu/healthsci/**

- **California:** ValleyCare Health Library & Ryan Comer Cancer Resource Center (ValleyCare Health System, Pleasanton), **http://gaelnet.stmarys-ca.edu/other.libs/gbal/east/vchl.html**

- **California:** Washington Community Health Resource Library (Fremont), **http://www.healthlibrary.org/**

- **Colorado:** William V. Gervasini Memorial Library (Exempla Healthcare), **http://www.saintjosephdenver.org/yourhealth/libraries/**

- **Connecticut:** Hartford Hospital Health Science Libraries (Hartford Hospital), **http://www.harthosp.org/library/**

- **Connecticut:** Healthnet: Connecticut Consumer Health Information Center (University of Connecticut Health Center, Lyman Maynard Stowe Library), **http://library.uchc.edu/departm/hnet/**

---

[18] Abstracted from **http://www.nlm.nih.gov/medlineplus/libraries.html**.

- **Connecticut:** Waterbury Hospital Health Center Library (Waterbury Hospital, Waterbury), **http://www.waterburyhospital.com/library/consumer.shtml**

- **Delaware:** Consumer Health Library (Christiana Care Health System, Eugene du Pont Preventive Medicine & Rehabilitation Institute, Wilmington), **http://www.christianacare.org/health_guide/health_guide_pmri_health_info.cfm**

- **Delaware:** Lewis B. Flinn Library (Delaware Academy of Medicine, Wilmington), **http://www.delamed.org/chls.html**

- **Georgia:** Family Resource Library (Medical College of Georgia, Augusta), **http://cmc.mcg.edu/kids_families/fam_resources/fam_res_lib/frl.htm**

- **Georgia:** Health Resource Center (Medical Center of Central Georgia, Macon), **http://www.mccg.org/hrc/hrchome.asp**

- **Hawaii:** Hawaii Medical Library: Consumer Health Information Service (Hawaii Medical Library, Honolulu), **http://hml.org/CHIS/**

- **Idaho:** DeArmond Consumer Health Library (Kootenai Medical Center, Coeur d'Alene), **http://www.nicon.org/DeArmond/index.htm**

- **Illinois:** Health Learning Center of Northwestern Memorial Hospital (Chicago), **http://www.nmh.org/health_info/hlc.html**

- **Illinois:** Medical Library (OSF Saint Francis Medical Center, Peoria), **http://www.osfsaintfrancis.org/general/library/**

- **Kentucky:** Medical Library - Services for Patients, Families, Students & the Public (Central Baptist Hospital, Lexington), **http://www.centralbap.com/education/community/library.cfm**

- **Kentucky:** University of Kentucky - Health Information Library (Chandler Medical Center, Lexington), **http://www.mc.uky.edu/PatientEd/**

- **Louisiana:** Alton Ochsner Medical Foundation Library (Alton Ochsner Medical Foundation, New Orleans), **http://www.ochsner.org/library/**

- **Louisiana:** Louisiana State University Health Sciences Center Medical Library-Shreveport, **http://lib-sh.lsuhsc.edu/**

- **Maine:** Franklin Memorial Hospital Medical Library (Franklin Memorial Hospital, Farmington), **http://www.fchn.org/fmh/lib.htm**

- **Maine:** Gerrish-True Health Sciences Library (Central Maine Medical Center, Lewiston), **http://www.cmmc.org/library/library.html**

- **Maine:** Hadley Parrot Health Science Library (Eastern Maine Healthcare, Bangor), **http://www.emh.org/hll/hpl/guide.htm**

- **Maine:** Maine Medical Center Library (Maine Medical Center, Portland), **http://www.mmc.org/library/**

- **Maine:** Parkview Hospital (Brunswick), **http://www.parkviewhospital.org/**

- **Maine:** Southern Maine Medical Center Health Sciences Library (Southern Maine Medical Center, Biddeford), **http://www.smmc.org/services/service.php3?choice=10**

- **Maine:** Stephens Memorial Hospital's Health Information Library (Western Maine Health, Norway), **http://www.wmhcc.org/Library/**

- **Manitoba, Canada:** Consumer & Patient Health Information Service (University of Manitoba Libraries), http://www.umanitoba.ca/libraries/units/health/reference/chis.html

- **Manitoba, Canada:** J.W. Crane Memorial Library (Deer Lodge Centre, Winnipeg), http://www.deerlodge.mb.ca/crane_library/about.asp

- **Maryland:** Health Information Center at the Wheaton Regional Library (Montgomery County, Dept. of Public Libraries, Wheaton Regional Library), http://www.mont.lib.md.us/healthinfo/hic.asp

- **Massachusetts:** Baystate Medical Center Library (Baystate Health System), http://www.baystatehealth.com/1024/

- **Massachusetts:** Boston University Medical Center Alumni Medical Library (Boston University Medical Center), http://med-libwww.bu.edu/library/lib.html

- **Massachusetts:** Lowell General Hospital Health Sciences Library (Lowell General Hospital, Lowell), http://www.lowellgeneral.org/library/HomePageLinks/WWW.htm

- **Massachusetts:** Paul E. Woodard Health Sciences Library (New England Baptist Hospital, Boston), http://www.nebh.org/health_lib.asp

- **Massachusetts:** St. Luke's Hospital Health Sciences Library (St. Luke's Hospital, Southcoast Health System, New Bedford), http://www.southcoast.org/library/

- **Massachusetts:** Treadwell Library Consumer Health Reference Center (Massachusetts General Hospital), http://www.mgh.harvard.edu/library/chrcindex.html

- **Massachusetts:** UMass HealthNet (University of Massachusetts Medical School, Worchester), http://healthnet.umassmed.edu/

- **Michigan:** Botsford General Hospital Library - Consumer Health (Botsford General Hospital, Library & Internet Services), http://www.botsfordlibrary.org/consumer.htm

- **Michigan:** Helen DeRoy Medical Library (Providence Hospital and Medical Centers), http://www.providence-hospital.org/library/

- **Michigan:** Marquette General Hospital - Consumer Health Library (Marquette General Hospital, Health Information Center), http://www.mgh.org/center.html

- **Michigan:** Patient Education Resouce Center - University of Michigan Cancer Center (University of Michigan Comprehensive Cancer Center, Ann Arbor), http://www.cancer.med.umich.edu/learn/leares.htm

- **Michigan:** Sladen Library & Center for Health Information Resources - Consumer Health Information (Detroit), http://www.henryford.com/body.cfm?id=39330

- **Montana:** Center for Health Information (St. Patrick Hospital and Health Sciences Center, Missoula)

- **National:** Consumer Health Library Directory (Medical Library Association, Consumer and Patient Health Information Section), http://caphis.mlanet.org/directory/index.html

- **National:** National Network of Libraries of Medicine (National Library of Medicine) - provides library services for health professionals in the United States who do not have access to a medical library, http://nnlm.gov/

- **National:** NN/LM List of Libraries Serving the Public (National Network of Libraries of Medicine), http://nnlm.gov/members/

- **Nevada:** Health Science Library, West Charleston Library (Las Vegas-Clark County Library District, Las Vegas), http://www.lvccld.org/special_collections/medical/index.htm

- **New Hampshire:** Dartmouth Biomedical Libraries (Dartmouth College Library, Hanover), http://www.dartmouth.edu/~biomed/resources.htmld/conshealth.htmld/

- **New Jersey:** Consumer Health Library (Rahway Hospital, Rahway), http://www.rahwayhospital.com/library.htm

- **New Jersey:** Dr. Walter Phillips Health Sciences Library (Englewood Hospital and Medical Center, Englewood), http://www.englewoodhospital.com/links/index.htm

- **New Jersey:** Meland Foundation (Englewood Hospital and Medical Center, Englewood), http://www.geocities.com/ResearchTriangle/9360/

- **New York:** Choices in Health Information (New York Public Library) - NLM Consumer Pilot Project participant, http://www.nypl.org/branch/health/links.html

- **New York:** Health Information Center (Upstate Medical University, State University of New York, Syracuse), http://www.upstate.edu/library/hic/

- **New York:** Health Sciences Library (Long Island Jewish Medical Center, New Hyde Park), http://www.lij.edu/library/library.html

- **New York:** ViaHealth Medical Library (Rochester General Hospital), http://www.nyam.org/library/

- **Ohio:** Consumer Health Library (Akron General Medical Center, Medical & Consumer Health Library), http://www.akrongeneral.org/hwlibrary.htm

- **Oklahoma:** The Health Information Center at Saint Francis Hospital (Saint Francis Health System, Tulsa), http://www.sfh-tulsa.com/services/healthinfo.asp

- **Oregon:** Planetree Health Resource Center (Mid-Columbia Medical Center, The Dalles), http://www.mcmc.net/phrc/

- **Pennsylvania:** Community Health Information Library (Milton S. Hershey Medical Center, Hershey), http://www.hmc.psu.edu/commhealth/

- **Pennsylvania:** Community Health Resource Library (Geisinger Medical Center, Danville), http://www.geisinger.edu/education/commlib.shtml

- **Pennsylvania:** HealthInfo Library (Moses Taylor Hospital, Scranton), http://www.mth.org/healthwellness.html

- **Pennsylvania:** Hopwood Library (University of Pittsburgh, Health Sciences Library System, Pittsburgh), http://www.hsls.pitt.edu/guides/chi/hopwood/index_html

- **Pennsylvania:** Koop Community Health Information Center (College of Physicians of Philadelphia), http://www.collphyphil.org/kooppg1.shtml

- **Pennsylvania:** Learning Resources Center - Medical Library (Susquehanna Health System, Williamsport), http://www.shscares.org/services/lrc/index.asp

- **Pennsylvania:** Medical Library (UPMC Health System, Pittsburgh), http://www.upmc.edu/passavant/library.htm

- **Quebec, Canada:** Medical Library (Montreal General Hospital), http://www.mghlib.mcgill.ca/

- **South Dakota:** Rapid City Regional Hospital Medical Library (Rapid City Regional Hospital), **http://www.rcrh.org/Services/Library/Default.asp**

- **Texas:** Houston HealthWays (Houston Academy of Medicine-Texas Medical Center Library), **http://hhw.library.tmc.edu/**

- **Washington:** Community Health Library (Kittitas Valley Community Hospital), **http://www.kvch.com/**

- **Washington:** Southwest Washington Medical Center Library (Southwest Washington Medical Center, Vancouver), **http://www.swmedicalcenter.com/body.cfm?id=72**

ONLINE GLOSSARIES

The Internet provides access to a number of free-to-use medical dictionaries. The National Library of Medicine has compiled the following list of online dictionaries:

- ADAM Medical Encyclopedia (A.D.A.M., Inc.), comprehensive medical reference: **http://www.nlm.nih.gov/medlineplus/encyclopedia.html**

- MedicineNet.com Medical Dictionary (MedicineNet, Inc.): **http://www.medterms.com/Script/Main/hp.asp**

- Merriam-Webster Medical Dictionary (Inteli-Health, Inc.): **http://www.intelihealth.com/IH/**

- Multilingual Glossary of Technical and Popular Medical Terms in Eight European Languages (European Commission) - Danish, Dutch, English, French, German, Italian, Portuguese, and Spanish: **http://allserv.rug.ac.be/~rvdstich/eugloss/welcome.html**

- On-line Medical Dictionary (CancerWEB): **http://cancerweb.ncl.ac.uk/omd/**

- Rare Diseases Terms (Office of Rare Diseases): **http://ord.aspensys.com/asp/diseases/diseases.asp**

- Technology Glossary (National Library of Medicine) - Health Care Technology: **http://www.nlm.nih.gov/nichsr/ta101/ta10108.htm**

Beyond these, MEDLINEplus contains a very patient-friendly encyclopedia covering every aspect of medicine (licensed from A.D.A.M., Inc.). The ADAM Medical Encyclopedia can be accessed at **http://www.nlm.nih.gov/medlineplus/encyclopedia.html**. ADAM is also available on commercial Web sites such as drkoop.com (**http://www.drkoop.com/**) and Web MD (**http://my.webmd.com/adam/asset/adam_disease_articles/a_to_z/a**). The NIH suggests the following Web sites in the ADAM Medical Encyclopedia when searching for information on essential tremor:

- **Basic Guidelines for Essential Tremor**

  Essential tremor
  Web site: http://www.nlm.nih.gov/medlineplus/ency/article/000762.htm

- **Signs & Symptoms for Essential Tremor**

  Confusion
  Web site: http://www.nlm.nih.gov/medlineplus/ency/article/003205.htm

  Fainting
  Web site: http://www.nlm.nih.gov/medlineplus/ency/article/003092.htm

  Nausea/vomiting
  Web site: http://www.nlm.nih.gov/medlineplus/ency/article/003117.htm

  Stress
  Web site: http://www.nlm.nih.gov/medlineplus/ency/article/003211.htm

- **Diagnostics and Tests for Essential Tremor**

  CT
  Web site: http://www.nlm.nih.gov/medlineplus/ency/article/003330.htm

  Head CT
  Web site: http://www.nlm.nih.gov/medlineplus/ency/article/003786.htm

  Head CT scan
  Web site: http://www.nlm.nih.gov/medlineplus/ency/article/003786.htm

  Heart rate
  Web site: http://www.nlm.nih.gov/medlineplus/ency/article/003399.htm

  MRI
  Web site: http://www.nlm.nih.gov/medlineplus/ency/article/003335.htm

  X-ray
  Web site: http://www.nlm.nih.gov/medlineplus/ency/article/003337.htm

- **Nutrition for Essential Tremor**

  Caffeine
  Web site: http://www.nlm.nih.gov/medlineplus/ency/article/002445.htm

  Coffee
  Web site: http://www.nlm.nih.gov/medlineplus/ency/article/002445.htm

- **Background Topics for Essential Tremor**

  Benign
  Web site: http://www.nlm.nih.gov/medlineplus/ency/article/002236.htm

  Stimulants
  Web site: http://www.nlm.nih.gov/medlineplus/ency/article/002308.htm

Online Dictionary Directories

The following are additional online directories compiled by the National Library of Medicine, including a number of specialized medical dictionaries:

- Medical Dictionaries: Medical & Biological (World Health Organization): **http://www.who.int/hlt/virtuallibrary/English/diction.htm#Medical**

- MEL-Michigan Electronic Library List of Online Health and Medical Dictionaries (Michigan Electronic Library): **http://mel.lib.mi.us/health/health-dictionaries.html**

- Patient Education: Glossaries (DMOZ Open Directory Project): **http://dmoz.org/Health/Education/Patient_Education/Glossaries/**

- Web of Online Dictionaries (Bucknell University): **http://www.yourdictionary.com/diction5.html#medicine**

ESSENTIAL TREMOR DICTIONARY

The definitions below are derived from official public sources, including the National Institutes of Health [NIH] and the European Union [EU].

Ablation: The removal of an organ by surgery. [NIH]

Acetylcholine: A neurotransmitter. Acetylcholine in vertebrates is the major transmitter at neuromuscular junctions, autonomic ganglia, parasympathetic effector junctions, a subset of sympathetic effector junctions, and at many sites in the central nervous system. It is generally not used as an administered drug because it is broken down very rapidly by cholinesterases, but it is useful in some ophthalmological applications. [NIH]

Activities of Daily Living: The performance of the basic activities of self care, such as dressing, ambulation, eating, etc., in rehabilitation. [NIH]

Adjunctive Therapy: Another treatment used together with the primary treatment. Its purpose is to assist the primary treatment. [NIH]

Adjuvant: A substance which aids another, such as an auxiliary remedy; in immunology, nonspecific stimulator (e.g., BCG vaccine) of the immune response. [EU]

Adrenaline: A hormone. Also called epinephrine. [NIH]

Adrenergic: Activated by, characteristic of, or secreting epinephrine or substances with similar activity; the term is applied to those nerve fibres that liberate norepinephrine at a synapse when a nerve impulse passes, i.e., the sympathetic fibres. [EU]

Adrenoreceptor: Receptors specifically sensitive to and operated by adrenaline and/or noradrenaline and related sympathomimetic drugs. Adrenoreceptor is an alternative name. [NIH]

Adverse Effect: An unwanted side effect of treatment. [NIH]

Afferent: Concerned with the transmission of neural impulse toward the central part of the nervous system. [NIH]

Affinity: 1. Inherent likeness or relationship. 2. A special attraction for a specific element, organ, or structure. 3. Chemical affinity; the force that binds atoms in molecules; the tendency of substances to combine by chemical reaction. 4. The strength of noncovalent chemical binding between two substances as measured by the dissociation constant of the complex. 5. In immunology, a thermodynamic expression of the strength of interaction between a single antigen-binding site and a single antigenic determinant (and thus of the stereochemical compatibility between them), most accurately applied to interactions among simple, uniform antigenic determinants such as haptens. Expressed as the association constant (K litres mole -1), which, owing to the heterogeneity of affinities in a population of antibody molecules of a given specificity, actually represents an average value (mean intrinsic association constant). 6. The reciprocal of the dissociation constant. [EU]

Age of Onset: The age or period of life at which a disease or the initial symptoms or manifestations of a disease appear in an individual. [NIH]

Agonist: In anatomy, a prime mover. In pharmacology, a drug that has affinity for and stimulates physiologic activity at cell receptors normally stimulated by naturally occurring substances. [EU]

Agoraphobia: Obsessive, persistent, intense fear of open places. [NIH]

Airway: A device for securing unobstructed passage of air into and out of the lungs during general anesthesia. [NIH]

Akathisia: 1. A condition of motor restlessness in which there is a feeling of muscular quivering, an urge to move about constantly, and an inability to sit still, a common extrapyramidal side effect of neuroleptic drugs. 2. An inability to sit down because of intense anxiety at the thought of doing so. [EU]

Akinesia: 1. Absence or poverty of movements. 2. The temporary paralysis of a muscle by the injection of procaine. [EU]

Albumin: 1. Any protein that is soluble in water and moderately concentrated salt solutions and is coagulable by heat. 2. Serum albumin; the major plasma protein (approximately 60 per cent of the total), which is responsible for much of the plasma colloidal osmotic pressure and serves as a transport protein carrying large organic anions, such as fatty acids, bilirubin, and many drugs, and also carrying certain hormones, such as cortisol and thyroxine, when their specific binding globulins are saturated. Albumin is synthesized in the liver. Low serum levels occur in protein malnutrition, active inflammation and serious hepatic and renal disease. [EU]

Algorithms: A procedure consisting of a sequence of algebraic formulas and/or logical steps to calculate or determine a given task. [NIH]

Alimentary: Pertaining to food or nutritive material, or to the organs of digestion. [EU]

Alleles: Mutually exclusive forms of the same gene, occupying the same locus on homologous chromosomes, and governing the same biochemical and developmental process. [NIH]

Alprenolol: 1-((1-Methylethyl)amino)-3-(2-(2-propenyl)phenoxy)-2-propanol. Adrenergic beta-blocker used as an antihypertensive, anti-anginal, and anti-arrhythmic agent. [NIH]

Alternative medicine: Practices not generally recognized by the medical community as standard or conventional medical approaches and used instead of standard treatments. Alternative medicine includes the taking of dietary supplements, megadose vitamins, and herbal preparations; the drinking of special teas; and practices such as massage therapy, magnet therapy, spiritual healing, and meditation. [NIH]

Amino acid: Any organic compound containing an amino (-NH2 and a carboxyl (- COOH) group. The 20 a-amino acids listed in the accompanying table are the amino acids from which proteins are synthesized by formation of peptide bonds during ribosomal translation of messenger RNA; all except glycine, which is not optically active, have the L configuration. Other amino acids occurring in proteins, such as hydroxyproline in collagen, are formed by posttranslational enzymatic modification of amino acids residues in polypeptide chains. There are also several important amino acids, such as the neurotransmitter y-aminobutyric acid, that have no relation to proteins. Abbreviated AA. [EU]

Amino Acid Sequence: The order of amino acids as they occur in a polypeptide chain. This is referred to as the primary structure of proteins. It is of fundamental importance in determining protein conformation. [NIH]

Amygdala: Almond-shaped group of basal nuclei anterior to the inferior horn of the lateral ventricle of the brain, within the temporal lobe. The amygdala is part of the limbic system. [NIH]

Anal: Having to do with the anus, which is the posterior opening of the large bowel. [NIH]

Analog: In chemistry, a substance that is similar, but not identical, to another. [NIH]

Anatomical: Pertaining to anatomy, or to the structure of the organism. [EU]

Anesthesia: A state characterized by loss of feeling or sensation. This depression of nerve function is usually the result of pharmacologic action and is induced to allow performance of surgery or other painful procedures. [NIH]

Angina: Chest pain that originates in the heart. [NIH]

Angina Pectoris: The symptom of paroxysmal pain consequent to myocardial ischemia usually of distinctive character, location and radiation, and provoked by a transient stressful situation during which the oxygen requirements of the myocardium exceed the capacity of the coronary circulation to supply it. [NIH]

Animal model: An animal with a disease either the same as or like a disease in humans. Animal models are used to study the development and progression of diseases and to test new treatments before they are given to humans. Animals with transplanted human cancers or other tissues are called xenograft models. [NIH]

Antagonism: Interference with, or inhibition of, the growth of a living organism by another living organism, due either to creation of unfavorable conditions (e. g. exhaustion of food supplies) or to production of a specific antibiotic substance (e. g. penicillin). [NIH]

Antibacterial: A substance that destroys bacteria or suppresses their growth or reproduction. [EU]

Antibiotic: A drug used to treat infections caused by bacteria and other microorganisms. [NIH]

Anticonvulsant: An agent that prevents or relieves convulsions. [EU]

Antiemetic: An agent that prevents or alleviates nausea and vomiting. Also antinauseant. [EU]

Antiepileptic: An agent that combats epilepsy. [EU]

Antipsychotic: Effective in the treatment of psychosis. Antipsychotic drugs (called also neuroleptic drugs and major tranquilizers) are a chemically diverse (including phenothiazines, thioxanthenes, butyrophenones, dibenzoxazepines, dibenzodiazepines, and diphenylbutylpiperidines) but pharmacologically similar class of drugs used to treat schizophrenic, paranoid, schizoaffective, and other psychotic disorders; acute delirium and dementia, and manic episodes (during induction of lithium therapy); to control the movement disorders associated with Huntington's chorea, Gilles de la Tourette's syndrome, and ballismus; and to treat intractable hiccups and severe nausea and vomiting. Antipsychotic agents bind to dopamine, histamine, muscarinic cholinergic, a-adrenergic, and serotonin receptors. Blockade of dopaminergic transmission in various areas is thought to be responsible for their major effects : antipsychotic action by blockade in the mesolimbic and mesocortical areas; extrapyramidal side effects (dystonia, akathisia, parkinsonism, and tardive dyskinesia) by blockade in the basal ganglia; and antiemetic effects by blockade in the chemoreceptor trigger zone of the medulla. Sedation and autonomic side effects (orthostatic hypotension, blurred vision, dry mouth, nasal congestion and constipation) are caused by blockade of histamine, cholinergic, and adrenergic receptors. [EU]

Anxiety: Persistent feeling of dread, apprehension, and impending disaster. [NIH]

Arterial: Pertaining to an artery or to the arteries. [EU]

Arteries: The vessels carrying blood away from the heart. [NIH]

Arterioles: The smallest divisions of the arteries located between the muscular arteries and the capillaries. [NIH]

Artery: Vessel-carrying blood from the heart to various parts of the body. [NIH]

Astringents: Agents, usually topical, that cause the contraction of tissues for the control of bleeding or secretions. [NIH]

Asymptomatic: Having no signs or symptoms of disease. [NIH]

Atenolol: A cardioselective beta-adrenergic blocker possessing properties and potency similar to propranolol, but without a negative inotropic effect. [NIH]

Atrial: Pertaining to an atrium. [EU]

Atrophy: Decrease in the size of a cell, tissue, organ, or multiple organs, associated with a variety of pathological conditions such as abnormal cellular changes, ischemia, malnutrition, or hormonal changes. [NIH]

Attenuation: Reduction of transmitted sound energy or its electrical equivalent. [NIH]

Atypical: Irregular; not conformable to the type; in microbiology, applied specifically to strains of unusual type. [EU]

Auditory: Pertaining to the sense of hearing. [EU]

Autoimmune disease: A condition in which the body recognizes its own tissues as foreign and directs an immune response against them. [NIH]

Autonomic: Self-controlling; functionally independent. [EU]

Autonomic Nervous System: The enteric, parasympathetic, and sympathetic nervous systems taken together. Generally speaking, the autonomic nervous system regulates the internal environment during both peaceful activity and physical or emotional stress. Autonomic activity is controlled and integrated by the central nervous system, especially the hypothalamus and the solitary nucleus, which receive information relayed from visceral afferents; these and related central and sensory structures are sometimes (but not here) considered to be part of the autonomic nervous system itself. [NIH]

Autopsy: Postmortem examination of the body. [NIH]

Axons: Nerve fibers that are capable of rapidly conducting impulses away from the neuron cell body. [NIH]

Bacteria: Unicellular prokaryotic microorganisms which generally possess rigid cell walls, multiply by cell division, and exhibit three principal forms: round or coccal, rodlike or bacillary, and spiral or spirochetal. [NIH]

Bactericidal: Substance lethal to bacteria; substance capable of killing bacteria. [NIH]

Basal Ganglia: Large subcortical nuclear masses derived from the telencephalon and located in the basal regions of the cerebral hemispheres. [NIH]

Basal Ganglia Diseases: Diseases of the basal ganglia including the putamen; globus pallidus; claustrum; amygdala; and caudate nucleus. Dyskinesias (most notably involuntary movements and alterations of the rate of movement) represent the primary clinical manifestations of these disorders. Common etiologies include cerebrovascular disease; neurodegenerative diseases; and craniocerebral trauma. [NIH]

Benign: Not cancerous; does not invade nearby tissue or spread to other parts of the body. [NIH]

Bilateral: Affecting both the right and left side of body. [NIH]

Biochemical: Relating to biochemistry; characterized by, produced by, or involving chemical reactions in living organisms. [EU]

Biomarkers: Substances sometimes found in an increased amount in the blood, other body fluids, or tissues and that may suggest the presence of some types of cancer. Biomarkers include CA 125 (ovarian cancer), CA 15-3 (breast cancer), CEA (ovarian, lung, breast, pancreas, and GI tract cancers), and PSA (prostate cancer). Also called tumor markers. [NIH]

Biotechnology: Body of knowledge related to the use of organisms, cells or cell-derived constituents for the purpose of developing products which are technically, scientifically and clinically useful. Alteration of biologic function at the molecular level (i.e., genetic engineering) is a central focus; laboratory methods used include transfection and cloning technologies, sequence and structure analysis algorithms, computer databases, and gene and protein structure function analysis and prediction. [NIH]

Bladder: The organ that stores urine. [NIH]

Blepharospasm: Excessive winking; tonic or clonic spasm of the orbicularis oculi muscle. [NIH]

Blood Platelets: Non-nucleated disk-shaped cells formed in the megakaryocyte and found in the blood of all mammals. They are mainly involved in blood coagulation. [NIH]

Blood vessel: A tube in the body through which blood circulates. Blood vessels include a network of arteries, arterioles, capillaries, venules, and veins. [NIH]

Blood-Brain Barrier: Specialized non-fenestrated tightly-joined endothelial cells (tight junctions) that form a transport barrier for certain substances between the cerebral capillaries and the brain tissue. [NIH]

Body Fluids: Liquid components of living organisms. [NIH]

Body Mass Index: One of the anthropometric measures of body mass; it has the highest correlation with skinfold thickness or body density. [NIH]

Bone Marrow: The soft tissue filling the cavities of bones. Bone marrow exists in two types, yellow and red. Yellow marrow is found in the large cavities of large bones and consists mostly of fat cells and a few primitive blood cells. Red marrow is a hematopoietic tissue and is the site of production of erythrocytes and granular leukocytes. Bone marrow is made up of a framework of connective tissue containing branching fibers with the frame being filled with marrow cells. [NIH]

Brachial: All the nerves from the arm are ripped from the spinal cord. [NIH]

Brachial Plexus: The large network of nerve fibers which distributes the innervation of the upper extremity. The brachial plexus extends from the neck into the axilla. In humans, the nerves of the plexus usually originate from the lower cervical and the first thoracic spinal cord segments (C5-C8 and T1), but variations are not uncommon. [NIH]

Brain Hypoxia: Lack of oxygen leading to unconsciousness. [NIH]

Brain Infarction: The formation of an area of necrosis in the brain, including the cerebral hemispheres (cerebral infarction), thalami, basal ganglia, brain stem (brain stem infarctions), or cerebellum secondary to an insufficiency of arterial or venous blood flow. [NIH]

Brain Ischemia: Localized reduction of blood flow to brain tissue due to arterial obtruction or systemic hypoperfusion. This frequently occurs in conjuction with brain hypoxia. Prolonged ischemia is associated with brain infarction. [NIH]

Brain Stem: The part of the brain that connects the cerebral hemispheres with the spinal cord. It consists of the mesencephalon, pons, and medulla oblongata. [NIH]

Bronchi: The larger air passages of the lungs arising from the terminal bifurcation of the trachea. [NIH]

Bronchodilator: A drug that relaxes the smooth muscles in the constricted airway. [NIH]

Butyric Acid: A four carbon acid, CH3CH2CH2COOH, with an unpleasant odor that occurs in butter and animal fat as the glycerol ester. [NIH]

Calcium: A basic element found in nearly all organized tissues. It is a member of the alkaline earth family of metals with the atomic symbol Ca, atomic number 20, and atomic weight 40. Calcium is the most abundant mineral in the body and combines with phosphorus to form calcium phosphate in the bones and teeth. It is essential for the normal functioning of nerves and muscles and plays a role in blood coagulation (as factor IV) and in many enzymatic processes. [NIH]

Calibration: Determination, by measurement or comparison with a standard, of the correct value of each scale reading on a meter or other measuring instrument; or determination of the settings of a control device that correspond to particular values of voltage, current, frequency, or other output. [NIH]

Calmodulin: A heat-stable, low-molecular-weight activator protein found mainly in the brain and heart. The binding of calcium ions to this protein allows this protein to bind to cyclic nucleotide phosphodiesterases and to adenyl cyclase with subsequent activation. Thereby this protein modulates cyclic AMP and cyclic GMP levels. [NIH]

Caloric intake: Refers to the number of calories (energy content) consumed. [NIH]

Carcinogenic: Producing carcinoma. [EU]

Cardiac: Having to do with the heart. [NIH]

Cardioselective: Having greater activity on heart tissue than on other tissue. [EU]

Cardiovascular: Having to do with the heart and blood vessels. [NIH]

Case report: A detailed report of the diagnosis, treatment, and follow-up of an individual patient. Case reports also contain some demographic information about the patient (for example, age, gender, ethnic origin). [NIH]

Case series: A group or series of case reports involving patients who were given similar treatment. Reports of case series usually contain detailed information about the individual patients. This includes demographic information (for example, age, gender, ethnic origin) and information on diagnosis, treatment, response to treatment, and follow-up after treatment. [NIH]

Causal: Pertaining to a cause; directed against a cause. [EU]

Cell: The individual unit that makes up all of the tissues of the body. All living things are made up of one or more cells. [NIH]

Cell membrane: Cell membrane = plasma membrane. The structure enveloping a cell, enclosing the cytoplasm, and forming a selective permeability barrier; it consists of lipids, proteins, and some carbohydrates, the lipids thought to form a bilayer in which integral proteins are embedded to varying degrees. [EU]

Central Nervous System: The main information-processing organs of the nervous system, consisting of the brain, spinal cord, and meninges. [NIH]

Cerebellar: Pertaining to the cerebellum. [EU]

Cerebellar Diseases: Diseases that affect the structure or function of the cerebellum. Cardinal manifestations of cerebellar dysfunction include dysmetria, gait ataxia, and muscle hypotonia. [NIH]

Cerebellum: Part of the metencephalon that lies in the posterior cranial fossa behind the brain stem. It is concerned with the coordination of movement. [NIH]

Cerebral: Of or pertaining of the cerebrum or the brain. [EU]

Cerebral Cortex: The thin layer of gray matter on the surface of the cerebral hemisphere that develops from the telencephalon and folds into gyri. It reaches its highest development in man and is responsible for intellectual faculties and higher mental functions. [NIH]

Cerebrum: The largest part of the brain. It is divided into two hemispheres, or halves, called the cerebral hemispheres. The cerebrum controls muscle functions of the body and also controls speech, emotions, reading, writing, and learning. [NIH]

Cervical: Relating to the neck, or to the neck of any organ or structure. Cervical lymph nodes are located in the neck; cervical cancer refers to cancer of the uterine cervix, which is the lower, narrow end (the "neck") of the uterus. [NIH]

Cervix: The lower, narrow end of the uterus that forms a canal between the uterus and vagina. [NIH]

Character: In current usage, approximately equivalent to personality. The sum of the relatively fixed personality traits and habitual modes of response of an individual. [NIH]

Chemoreceptor: A receptor adapted for excitation by chemical substances, e.g., olfactory and gustatory receptors, or a sense organ, as the carotid body or the aortic (supracardial) bodies, which is sensitive to chemical changes in the blood stream, especially reduced oxygen content, and reflexly increases both respiration and blood pressure. [EU]

Chin: The anatomical frontal portion of the mandible, also known as the mentum, that contains the line of fusion of the two separate halves of the mandible (symphysis menti). This line of fusion divides inferiorly to enclose a triangular area called the mental protuberance. On each side, inferior to the second premolar tooth, is the mental foramen for the passage of blood vessels and a nerve. [NIH]

Chlorpyrifos: An organothiophosphate cholinesterase inhibitor that is used as an insecticide and as an acaricide. [NIH]

Cholinergic: Resembling acetylcholine in pharmacological action; stimulated by or releasing acetylcholine or a related compound. [EU]

Chorea: Involuntary, forcible, rapid, jerky movements that may be subtle or become confluent, markedly altering normal patterns of movement. Hypotonia and pendular reflexes are often associated. Conditions which feature recurrent or persistent episodes of chorea as a primary manifestation of disease are referred to as choreatic disorders. Chorea is also a frequent manifestation of basal ganglia diseases. [NIH]

Choreatic Disorders: Acquired and hereditary conditions which feature chorea as a primary manifestation of the disease process. [NIH]

Chromosome: Part of a cell that contains genetic information. Except for sperm and eggs, all human cells contain 46 chromosomes. [NIH]

Chronic: A disease or condition that persists or progresses over a long period of time. [NIH]

Clinical study: A research study in which patients receive treatment in a clinic or other medical facility. Reports of clinical studies can contain results for single patients (case reports) or many patients (case series or clinical trials). [NIH]

Clinical trial: A research study that tests how well new medical treatments or other interventions work in people. Each study is designed to test new methods of screening, prevention, diagnosis, or treatment of a disease. [NIH]

Clonazepam: An anticonvulsant used for several types of seizures, including myotonic or atonic seizures, photosensitive epilepsy, and absence seizures, although tolerance may develop. It is seldom effective in generalized tonic-clonic or partial seizures. The mechanism of action appears to involve the enhancement of gaba receptor responses. [NIH]

Clonic: Pertaining to or of the nature of clonus. [EU]

Cloning: The production of a number of genetically identical individuals; in genetic engineering, a process for the efficient replication of a great number of identical DNA molecules. [NIH]

Clozapine: A tricyclic dibenzodiazepine, classified as an atypical antipsychotic agent. It binds several types of central nervous system receptors, and displays a unique pharmacological profile. Clozapine is a serotonin antagonist, with strong binding to 5-HT 2A/2C receptor subtype. It also displays strong affinity to several dopaminergic receptors, but shows only weak antagonism at the dopamine D2 receptor, a receptor commonly thought to modulate neuroleptic activity. Agranulocytosis is a major adverse effect associated with administration of this agent. [NIH]

Cognition: Intellectual or mental process whereby an organism becomes aware of or obtains knowledge. [NIH]

Cohort Studies: Studies in which subsets of a defined population are identified. These groups may or may not be exposed to factors hypothesized to influence the probability of the occurrence of a particular disease or other outcome. Cohorts are defined populations which, as a whole, are followed in an attempt to determine distinguishing subgroup characteristics. [NIH]

Complement: A term originally used to refer to the heat-labile factor in serum that causes immune cytolysis, the lysis of antibody-coated cells, and now referring to the entire functionally related system comprising at least 20 distinct serum proteins that is the effector not only of immune cytolysis but also of other biologic functions. Complement activation occurs by two different sequences, the classic and alternative pathways. The proteins of the classic pathway are termed 'components of complement' and are designated by the symbols C1 through C9. C1 is a calcium-dependent complex of three distinct proteins C1q, C1r and C1s. The proteins of the alternative pathway (collectively referred to as the properdin system) and complement regulatory proteins are known by semisystematic or trivial names. Fragments resulting from proteolytic cleavage of complement proteins are designated with lower-case letter suffixes, e.g., C3a. Inactivated fragments may be designated with the suffix 'i', e.g. C3bi. Activated components or complexes with biological activity are designated by a bar over the symbol e.g. C1 or C4b,2a. The classic pathway is activated by the binding of C1 to classic pathway activators, primarily antigen-antibody complexes containing IgM, IgG1, IgG3; C1q binds to a single IgM molecule or two adjacent IgG molecules. The alternative pathway can be activated by IgA immune complexes and also by nonimmunologic materials including bacterial endotoxins, microbial polysaccharides, and cell walls. Activation of the classic pathway triggers an enzymatic cascade involving C1, C4, C2 and C3; activation of the alternative pathway triggers a cascade involving C3 and factors B, D and P. Both result in the cleavage of C5 and the formation of the membrane attack complex. Complement activation also results in the formation of many biologically active complement fragments that act as anaphylatoxins, opsonins, or chemotactic factors. [EU]

Complementary and alternative medicine: CAM. Forms of treatment that are used in addition to (complementary) or instead of (alternative) standard treatments. These practices are not considered standard medical approaches. CAM includes dietary supplements, megadose vitamins, herbal preparations, special teas, massage therapy, magnet therapy, spiritual healing, and meditation. [NIH]

Complementary medicine: Practices not generally recognized by the medical community as standard or conventional medical approaches and used to enhance or complement the standard treatments. Complementary medicine includes the taking of dietary supplements, megadose vitamins, and herbal preparations; the drinking of special teas; and practices such as massage therapy, magnet therapy, spiritual healing, and meditation. [NIH]

Compress: A plug used to occlude an orifice in the control of bleeding, or to mop up secretions; an absorbent pad. [NIH]

Compulsions: In psychology, an irresistible urge, sometimes amounting to obsession to perform a particular act which usually is carried out against the performer's will or better judgment. [NIH]

Computational Biology: A field of biology concerned with the development of techniques for the collection and manipulation of biological data, and the use of such data to make biological discoveries or predictions. This field encompasses all computational methods and theories applicable to molecular biology and areas of computer-based techniques for solving biological problems including manipulation of models and datasets. [NIH]

Computer Systems: Systems composed of a computer or computers, peripheral equipment, such as disks, printers, and terminals, and telecommunications capabilities. [NIH]

Conduction: The transfer of sound waves, heat, nervous impulses, or electricity. [EU]

Congestion: Excessive or abnormal accumulation of blood in a part. [EU]

Conjunctiva: The mucous membrane that lines the inner surface of the eyelids and the anterior part of the sclera. [NIH]

Connective Tissue: Tissue that supports and binds other tissues. It consists of connective tissue cells embedded in a large amount of extracellular matrix. [NIH]

Connective Tissue: Tissue that supports and binds other tissues. It consists of connective tissue cells embedded in a large amount of extracellular matrix. [NIH]

Connexins: A group of homologous proteins which form the intermembrane channels of gap junctions. The connexins are the products of an identified gene family which has both highly conserved and highly divergent regions. The variety contributes to the wide range of functional properties of gap junctions. [NIH]

Consciousness: Sense of awareness of self and of the environment. [NIH]

Constipation: Infrequent or difficult evacuation of feces. [NIH]

Constriction: The act of constricting. [NIH]

Contracture: A condition of fixed high resistance to passive stretch of a muscle, resulting from fibrosis of the tissues supporting the muscles or the joints, or from disorders of the muscle fibres. [EU]

Contraindications: Any factor or sign that it is unwise to pursue a certain kind of action or treatment, e. g. giving a general anesthetic to a person with pneumonia. [NIH]

Contralateral: Having to do with the opposite side of the body. [NIH]

Controlled study: An experiment or clinical trial that includes a comparison (control) group. [NIH]

Convulsions: A general term referring to sudden and often violent motor activity of cerebral or brainstem origin. Convulsions may also occur in the absence of an electrical cerebral discharge (e.g., in response to hypotension). [NIH]

Convulsive: Relating or referring to spasm; affected with spasm; characterized by a spasm or spasms. [NIH]

Coordination: Muscular or motor regulation or the harmonious cooperation of muscles or groups of muscles, in a complex action or series of actions. [NIH]

Cornea: The transparent part of the eye that covers the iris and the pupil and allows light to enter the inside. [NIH]

Coronary: Encircling in the manner of a crown; a term applied to vessels; nerves, ligaments, etc. The term usually denotes the arteries that supply the heart muscle and, by extension, a pathologic involvement of them. [EU]

Coronary Thrombosis: Presence of a thrombus in a coronary artery, often causing a myocardial infarction. [NIH]

Corpus: The body of the uterus. [NIH]

Corpus Striatum: Striped gray and white matter consisting of the neostriatum and paleostriatum (globus pallidus). It is located in front of and lateral to the thalamus in each cerebral hemisphere. The gray substance is made up of the caudate nucleus and the lentiform nucleus (the latter consisting of the globus pallidus and putamen). The white matter is the internal capsule. [NIH]

Cortex: The outer layer of an organ or other body structure, as distinguished from the internal substance. [EU]

Cortical: Pertaining to or of the nature of a cortex or bark. [EU]

Cortices: The outer layer of an organ; used especially of the cerebrum and cerebellum. [NIH]

Cranial: Pertaining to the cranium, or to the anterior (in animals) or superior (in humans) end of the body. [EU]

Cross-Sectional Studies: Studies in which the presence or absence of disease or other health-related variables are determined in each member of the study population or in a representative sample at one particular time. This contrasts with longitudinal studies which are followed over a period of time. [NIH]

Curative: Tending to overcome disease and promote recovery. [EU]

Decarboxylation: The removal of a carboxyl group, usually in the form of carbon dioxide, from a chemical compound. [NIH]

Degenerative: Undergoing degeneration : tending to degenerate; having the character of or involving degeneration; causing or tending to cause degeneration. [EU]

Delirium: (DSM III-R) an acute, reversible organic mental disorder characterized by reduced ability to maintain attention to external stimuli and disorganized thinking as manifested by rambling, irrelevant, or incoherent speech; there are also a reduced level of consciousness, sensory misperceptions, disturbance of the sleep-wakefulness cycle and level of psychomotor activity, disorientation to time, place, or person, and memory impairment. Delirium may be caused by a large number of conditions resulting in derangement of cerebral metabolism, including systemic infection, poisoning, drug intoxication or withdrawal, seizures or head trauma, and metabolic disturbances such as hypoxia, hypoglycaemia, fluid, electrolyte, or acid-base imbalances, or hepatic or renal failure. Called also acute confusional state and acute brain syndrome. [EU]

Dementia: An acquired organic mental disorder with loss of intellectual abilities of sufficient severity to interfere with social or occupational functioning. The dysfunction is multifaceted and involves memory, behavior, personality, judgment, attention, spatial relations, language, abstract thought, and other executive functions. The intellectual decline is usually progressive, and initially spares the level of consciousness. [NIH]

Dendrites: Extensions of the nerve cell body. They are short and branched and receive stimuli from other neurons. [NIH]

Dendritic: 1. Branched like a tree. 2. Pertaining to or possessing dendrites. [EU]

Density: The logarithm to the base 10 of the opacity of an exposed and processed film. [NIH]

Depressive Disorder: An affective disorder manifested by either a dysphoric mood or loss of interest or pleasure in usual activities. The mood disturbance is prominent and relatively persistent. [NIH]

Diagnostic procedure: A method used to identify a disease. [NIH]

Diazinon: A cholinesterase inhibitor that is used as an organothiophosphorus insecticide. [NIH]

Diencephalon: The paired caudal parts of the prosencephalon from which the thalamus, hypothalamus, epithalamus, and subthalamus are derived. [NIH]

Direct: 1. Straight; in a straight line. 2. Performed immediately and without the intervention of subsidiary means. [EU]

Discrete: Made up of separate parts or characterized by lesions which do not become blended; not running together; separate. [NIH]

Disinfectant: An agent that disinfects; applied particularly to agents used on inanimate objects. [EU]

Distal: Remote; farther from any point of reference; opposed to proximal. In dentistry, used to designate a position on the dental arch farther from the median line of the jaw. [EU]

Diuretic: A drug that increases the production of urine. [NIH]

Dizziness: An imprecise term which may refer to a sense of spatial disorientation, motion of the environment, or lightheadedness. [NIH]

Dopa: The racemic or DL form of DOPA, an amino acid found in various legumes. The dextro form has little physiologic activity but the levo form (levodopa) is a very important physiologic mediator and precursor and pharmacological agent. [NIH]

Dopamine: An endogenous catecholamine and prominent neurotransmitter in several systems of the brain. In the synthesis of catecholamines from tyrosine, it is the immediate precursor to norepinephrine and epinephrine. Dopamine is a major transmitter in the extrapyramidal system of the brain, and important in regulating movement. A family of dopaminergic receptor subtypes mediate its action. Dopamine is used pharmacologically for its direct (beta adrenergic agonist) and indirect (adrenergic releasing) sympathomimetic effects including its actions as an inotropic agent and as a renal vasodilator. [NIH]

Double-blind: Pertaining to a clinical trial or other experiment in which neither the subject nor the person administering treatment knows which treatment any particular subject is receiving. [EU]

Drug Interactions: The action of a drug that may affect the activity, metabolism, or toxicity of another drug. [NIH]

Dyskinesia: Impairment of the power of voluntary movement, resulting in fragmentary or incomplete movements. [EU]

Dysphonia: Difficulty or pain in speaking; impairment of the voice. [NIH]

Dystrophy: Any disorder arising from defective or faulty nutrition, especially the muscular dystrophies. [EU]

Edema: Excessive amount of watery fluid accumulated in the intercellular spaces, most commonly present in subcutaneous tissue. [NIH]

Effector: It is often an enzyme that converts an inactive precursor molecule into an active second messenger. [NIH]

Efferent: Nerve fibers which conduct impulses from the central nervous system to muscles and glands. [NIH]

Efficacy: The extent to which a specific intervention, procedure, regimen, or service produces a beneficial result under ideal conditions. Ideally, the determination of efficacy is based on the results of a randomized control trial. [NIH]

Elective: Subject to the choice or decision of the patient or physician; applied to procedures that are advantageous to the patient but not urgent. [EU]

Electrode: Component of the pacing system which is at the distal end of the lead. It is the interface with living cardiac tissue across which the stimulus is transmitted. [NIH]

Electrons: Stable elementary particles having the smallest known negative charge, present in all elements; also called negatrons. Positively charged electrons are called positrons. The numbers, energies and arrangement of electrons around atomic nuclei determine the chemical identities of elements. Beams of electrons are called cathode rays or beta rays, the latter being a high-energy biproduct of nuclear decay. [NIH]

Electrophysiological: Pertaining to electrophysiology, that is a branch of physiology that is concerned with the electric phenomena associated with living bodies and involved in their functional activity. [EU]

Electroshock: Induction of a stress reaction in experimental subjects by means of an electrical shock; applies to either convulsive or non-convulsive states. [NIH]

Elementary Particles: Individual components of atoms, usually subatomic; subnuclear particles are usually detected only when the atomic nucleus decays and then only transiently, as most of them are unstable, often yielding pure energy without substance, i.e., radiation. [NIH]

Embolus: Bit of foreign matter which enters the blood stream at one point and is carried until it is lodged or impacted in an artery and obstructs it. It may be a blood clot, an air bubble, fat or other tissue, or clumps of bacteria. [NIH]

Endemic: Present or usually prevalent in a population or geographical area at all times; said of a disease or agent. Called also endemial. [EU]

Endorphins: One of the three major groups of endogenous opioid peptides. They are large peptides derived from the pro-opiomelanocortin precursor. The known members of this group are alpha-, beta-, and gamma-endorphin. The term endorphin is also sometimes used to refer to all opioid peptides, but the narrower sense is used here; opioid peptides is used for the broader group. [NIH]

Enkephalins: One of the three major families of endogenous opioid peptides. The enkephalins are pentapeptides that are widespread in the central and peripheral nervous systems and in the adrenal medulla. [NIH]

Environmental Exposure: The exposure to potentially harmful chemical, physical, or biological agents in the environment or to environmental factors that may include ionizing radiation, pathogenic organisms, or toxic chemicals. [NIH]

Environmental Health: The science of controlling or modifying those conditions, influences, or forces surrounding man which relate to promoting, establishing, and maintaining health. [NIH]

Enzyme: A protein that speeds up chemical reactions in the body. [NIH]

Epidemic: Occurring suddenly in numbers clearly in excess of normal expectancy; said especially of infectious diseases but applied also to any disease, injury, or other health-related event occurring in such outbreaks. [EU]

Epidemiologic Studies: Studies designed to examine associations, commonly, hypothesized causal relations. They are usually concerned with identifying or measuring the effects of risk factors or exposures. The common types of analytic study are case-control studies, cohort studies, and cross-sectional studies. [NIH]

Epidemiological: Relating to, or involving epidemiology. [EU]

Epinephrine: The active sympathomimetic hormone from the adrenal medulla in most species. It stimulates both the alpha- and beta- adrenergic systems, causes systemic vasoconstriction and gastrointestinal relaxation, stimulates the heart, and dilates bronchi and cerebral vessels. It is used in asthma and cardiac failure and to delay absorption of local anesthetics. [NIH]

Esotropia: A form of ocular misalignment characterized by an excessive convergence of the visual axes, resulting in a "cross-eye" appearance. An example of this condition occurs when paralysis of the lateral rectus muscle causes an abnormal inward deviation of one eye on attempted gaze. [NIH]

Essential Tremor: A rhythmic, involuntary, purposeless, oscillating movement resulting from the alternate contraction and relaxation of opposing groups of muscles. [NIH]

Ethanol: A clear, colorless liquid rapidly absorbed from the gastrointestinal tract and distributed throughout the body. It has bactericidal activity and is used often as a topical disinfectant. It is widely used as a solvent and preservative in pharmaceutical preparations as well as serving as the primary ingredient in alcoholic beverages. [NIH]

Evoke: The electric response recorded from the cerebral cortex after stimulation of a peripheral sense organ. [NIH]

Excitability: Property of a cardiac cell whereby, when the cell is depolarized to a critical level (called threshold), the membrane becomes permeable and a regenerative inward current causes an action potential. [NIH]

Excitation: An act of irritation or stimulation or of responding to a stimulus; the addition of energy, as the excitation of a molecule by absorption of photons. [EU]

Exon: The part of the DNA that encodes the information for the actual amino acid sequence of the protein. In many eucaryotic genes, the coding sequences consist of a series of exons alternating with intron sequences. [NIH]

Exotropia: A form of ocular misalignment where the visual axes diverge inappropriately. For example, medial rectus muscle weakness may produce this condition as the affected eye will deviate laterally upon attempted forward gaze. An exotropia occurs due to the relatively unopposed force exerted on the eye by the lateral rectus muscle, which pulls the eye in an outward direction. [NIH]

Expiratory: The volume of air which leaves the breathing organs in each expiration. [NIH]

Extrapyramidal: Outside of the pyramidal tracts. [EU]

Extremity: A limb; an arm or leg (membrum); sometimes applied specifically to a hand or foot. [EU]

Facial: Of or pertaining to the face. [EU]

Family Planning: Programs or services designed to assist the family in controlling reproduction by either improving or diminishing fertility. [NIH]

Fat: Total lipids including phospholipids. [NIH]

Fatigue: The state of weariness following a period of exertion, mental or physical, characterized by a decreased capacity for work and reduced efficiency to respond to stimuli. [NIH]

Fetus: The developing offspring from 7 to 8 weeks after conception until birth. [NIH]

Fibrosis: Any pathological condition where fibrous connective tissue invades any organ, usually as a consequence of inflammation or other injury. [NIH]

Fissure: Any cleft or groove, normal or otherwise; especially a deep fold in the cerebral cortex which involves the entire thickness of the brain wall. [EU]

Flunarizine: Flunarizine is a selective calcium entry blocker with calmodulin binding properties and histamine H1 blocking activity. It is effective in the prophylaxis of migraine, occlusive peripheral vascular disease, vertigo of central and peripheral origin, and as an adjuvant in the therapy of epilepsy. [NIH]

Fold: A plication or doubling of various parts of the body. [NIH]

Forearm: The part between the elbow and the wrist. [NIH]

Fossa: A cavity, depression, or pit. [NIH]

Frontal Lobe: The anterior part of the cerebral hemisphere. [NIH]

Functional magnetic resonance imaging: A noninvasive tool used to observe functioning in the brain or other organs by detecting changes in chemical composition, blood flow, or both. [NIH]

GABA: The most common inhibitory neurotransmitter in the central nervous system. [NIH]

Gait: Manner or style of walking. [NIH]

Gamma knife: Radiation therapy in which high-energy rays are aimed at a tumor from many angles in a single treatment session. [NIH]

Ganglia: Clusters of multipolar neurons surrounded by a capsule of loosely organized connective tissue located outside the central nervous system. [NIH]

Gap Junctions: Connections between cells which allow passage of small molecules and electric current. Gap junctions were first described anatomically as regions of close apposition between cells with a narrow (1-2 nm) gap between cell membranes. The variety in the properties of gap junctions is reflected in the number of connexins, the family of proteins which form the junctions. [NIH]

Gas: Air that comes from normal breakdown of food. The gases are passed out of the body through the rectum (flatus) or the mouth (burp). [NIH]

Gastrin: A hormone released after eating. Gastrin causes the stomach to produce more acid. [NIH]

Gastrointestinal: Refers to the stomach and intestines. [NIH]

Gastrointestinal tract: The stomach and intestines. [NIH]

Gene: The functional and physical unit of heredity passed from parent to offspring. Genes are pieces of DNA, and most genes contain the information for making a specific protein. [NIH]

Gene Expression: The phenotypic manifestation of a gene or genes by the processes of gene action. [NIH]

Gene Therapy: The introduction of new genes into cells for the purpose of treating disease by restoring or adding gene expression. Techniques include insertion of retroviral vectors, transfection, homologous recombination, and injection of new genes into the nuclei of single cell embryos. The entire gene therapy process may consist of multiple steps. The new genes may be introduced into proliferating cells in vivo (e.g., bone marrow) or in vitro (e.g., fibroblast cultures) and the modified cells transferred to the site where the gene expression is required. Gene therapy may be particularly useful for treating enzyme deficiency diseases, hemoglobinopathies, and leukemias and may also prove useful in restoring drug sensitivity, particularly for leukemia. [NIH]

Genetic Engineering: Directed modification of the gene complement of a living organism by such techniques as altering the DNA, substituting genetic material by means of a virus, transplanting whole nuclei, transplanting cell hybrids, etc. [NIH]

Genetics: The biological science that deals with the phenomena and mechanisms of heredity. [NIH]

Genotype: The genetic constitution of the individual; the characterization of the genes. [NIH]

Geriatric: Pertaining to the treatment of the aged. [EU]

Gland: An organ that produces and releases one or more substances for use in the body. Some glands produce fluids that affect tissues or organs. Others produce hormones or participate in blood production. [NIH]

Globus Pallidus: The representation of the phylogenetically oldest part of the corpus striatum called the paleostriatum. It forms the smaller, more medial part of the lentiform nucleus. [NIH]

Glutamate: Excitatory neurotransmitter of the brain. [NIH]

Glutamic Acid: A non-essential amino acid naturally occurring in the L-form. Glutamic acid (glutamate) is the most common excitatory neurotransmitter in the central nervous system. [NIH]

Glycerol: A trihydroxy sugar alcohol that is an intermediate in carbohydrate and lipid metabolism. It is used as a solvent, emollient, pharmaceutical agent, and sweetening agent. [NIH]

Glycine: A non-essential amino acid. It is found primarily in gelatin and silk fibroin and used therapeutically as a nutrient. It is also a fast inhibitory neurotransmitter. [NIH]

Governing Board: The group in which legal authority is vested for the control of health-related institutions and organizations. [NIH]

Grafting: The operation of transfer of tissue from one site to another. [NIH]

Hammer: The largest of the three ossicles of the ear. [NIH]

Haplotypes: The genetic constitution of individuals with respect to one member of a pair of allelic genes, or sets of genes that are closely linked and tend to be inherited together such as those of the major histocompatibility complex. [NIH]

Harmine: Alkaloid isolated from seeds of Peganum harmala L., Zygophyllaceae. It is identical to banisterine, or telepathine, from Banisteria caapi and is one of the active ingredients of hallucinogenic drinks made in the western Amazon region from related plants. It has no therapeutic use, but (as banisterine) was hailed as a cure for postencephalitic Parkinson disease in the 1920's. [NIH]

Hematoma: An extravasation of blood localized in an organ, space, or tissue. [NIH]

Hemoglobinopathies: A group of inherited disorders characterized by structural alterations within the hemoglobin molecule. [NIH]

Hemorrhage: Bleeding or escape of blood from a vessel. [NIH]

Hemorrhagic stroke: A disorder involving bleeding within ischemic brain tissue. Hemorrhagic stroke occurs when blood vessels that are damaged or dead from lack of blood supply (infarcted), located within an area of infarcted brain tissue, rupture and transform an "ischemic" stroke into a hemorrhagic stroke. Ischemia is inadequate tissue oxygenation caused by reduced blood flow; infarction is tissue death resulting from ischemia. Bleeding irritates the brain tissues, causing swelling (cerebral edema). Blood collects into a mass (hematoma). Both swelling and hematoma will compress and displace brain tissue. [NIH]

Hemostasis: The process which spontaneously arrests the flow of blood from vessels carrying blood under pressure. It is accomplished by contraction of the vessels, adhesion and aggregation of formed blood elements, and the process of blood or plasma coagulation. [NIH]

Hereditary: Of, relating to, or denoting factors that can be transmitted genetically from one generation to another. [NIH]

Heredity: 1. The genetic transmission of a particular quality or trait from parent to offspring. 2. The genetic constitution of an individual. [EU]

Heterogeneity: The property of one or more samples or populations which implies that they are not identical in respect of some or all of their parameters, e. g. heterogeneity of variance. [NIH]

Heterogenic: Derived from a different source or species. Also called heterogenous. [NIH]

Heterogenous: Derived from a different source or species. Also called heterogenic. [NIH]

Heterotropia: One in which the angle of squint remains relatively unaltered on conjugate movement of the eyes. [NIH]

Histamine: 1H-Imidazole-4-ethanamine. A depressor amine derived by enzymatic decarboxylation of histidine. It is a powerful stimulant of gastric secretion, a constrictor of bronchial smooth muscle, a vasodilator, and also a centrally acting neurotransmitter. [NIH]

Holidays: Days commemorating events. Holidays also include vacation periods. [NIH]

Homologous: Corresponding in structure, position, origin, etc., as (a) the feathers of a bird and the scales of a fish, (b) antigen and its specific antibody, (c) allelic chromosomes. [EU]

Hormone: A substance in the body that regulates certain organs. Hormones such as gastrin help in breaking down food. Some hormones come from cells in the stomach and small intestine. [NIH]

Hydration: Combining with water. [NIH]

Hypertension: Persistently high arterial blood pressure. Currently accepted threshold levels are 140 mm Hg systolic and 90 mm Hg diastolic pressure. [NIH]

Hyperthyroidism: Excessive functional activity of the thyroid gland. [NIH]

Hypokinesia: Slow or diminished movement of body musculature. It may be associated with basal ganglia diseases; mental disorders; prolonged inactivity due to illness; experimental protocols used to evaluate the physiologic effects of immobility; and other conditions. [NIH]

Hypotension: Abnormally low blood pressure. [NIH]

Ibotenic Acid: Neurotoxic isoxazole substance found in Amanita muscaria and A. pantherina. It causes motor depression, ataxia, and changes in mood, perceptions and feelings, and is a potent excitatory amino acid agonist. [NIH]

Idiopathic: Describes a disease of unknown cause. [NIH]

Illusion: A false interpretation of a genuine percept. [NIH]

Impairment: In the context of health experience, an impairment is any loss or abnormality of psychological, physiological, or anatomical structure or function. [NIH]

Implantation: The insertion or grafting into the body of biological, living, inert, or radioactive material. [EU]

In vitro: In the laboratory (outside the body). The opposite of in vivo (in the body). [NIH]

In vivo: In the body. The opposite of in vitro (outside the body or in the laboratory). [NIH]

Incision: A cut made in the body during surgery. [NIH]

Induction: The act or process of inducing or causing to occur, especially the production of a specific morphogenetic effect in the developing embryo through the influence of evocators or organizers, or the production of anaesthesia or unconsciousness by use of appropriate agents. [EU]

Infancy: The period of complete dependency prior to the acquisition of competence in walking, talking, and self-feeding. [NIH]

Infarction: A pathological process consisting of a sudden insufficient blood supply to an area, which results in necrosis of that area. It is usually caused by a thrombus, an embolus, or a vascular torsion. [NIH]

Infusion: A method of putting fluids, including drugs, into the bloodstream. Also called intravenous infusion. [NIH]

Ingestion: Taking into the body by mouth [NIH]

Inhalation: The drawing of air or other substances into the lungs. [EU]

Initiation: Mutation induced by a chemical reactive substance causing cell changes; being a step in a carcinogenic process. [NIH]

Innervation: 1. The distribution or supply of nerves to a part. 2. The supply of nervous energy or of nerve stimulus sent to a part. [EU]

Inotropic: Affecting the force or energy of muscular contractions. [EU]

Insecticides: Pesticides designed to control insects that are harmful to man. The insects may be directly harmful, as those acting as disease vectors, or indirectly harmful, as destroyers of crops, food products, or textile fabrics. [NIH]

Insulator: Material covering the metal conductor of the lead. It is usually polyurethane or silicone. [NIH]

Intervertebral: Situated between two contiguous vertebrae. [EU]

Intervertebral Disk Displacement: An intervertebral disk in which the nucleus pulposus has protruded through surrounding fibrocartilage. This occurs most frequently in the lower lumbar region. [NIH]

Intravenous: IV. Into a vein. [NIH]

Intrinsic: Situated entirely within or pertaining exclusively to a part. [EU]

Invasive: 1. Having the quality of invasiveness. 2. Involving puncture or incision of the skin or insertion of an instrument or foreign material into the body; said of diagnostic techniques. [EU]

Involuntary: Reaction occurring without intention or volition. [NIH]

Ionizing: Radiation comprising charged particles, e. g. electrons, protons, alpha-particles, etc., having sufficient kinetic energy to produce ionization by collision. [NIH]

Ischemia: Deficiency of blood in a part, due to functional constriction or actual obstruction of a blood vessel. [EU]

Isoniazid: Antibacterial agent used primarily as a tuberculostatic. It remains the treatment of choice for tuberculosis. [NIH]

Isoproterenol: Isopropyl analog of epinephrine; beta-sympathomimetic that acts on the heart, bronchi, skeletal muscle, alimentary tract, etc. It is used mainly as bronchodilator and heart stimulant. [NIH]

Kava: Dried rhizome and roots of Piper methysticum, a shrub native to Oceania and known for its anti-anxiety and sedative properties. Heavy usage results in some adverse effects. It contains alkaloids, lactones, kawain, methysticin, mucilage, starch, and yangonin. Kava is also the name of the pungent beverage prepared from the plant's roots. [NIH]

Kb: A measure of the length of DNA fragments, 1 Kb = 1000 base pairs. The largest DNA fragments are up to 50 kilobases long. [NIH]

Kinetic: Pertaining to or producing motion. [EU]

Lag: The time elapsing between application of a stimulus and the resulting reaction. [NIH]

Laryngeal: Having to do with the larynx. [NIH]

Laryngeal Muscles: The intrinsic muscles of the larynx are the aryepiglottic(us), arytenoid(eus), cricoarytenoid(eus), cricothyroid(eus), thyroarytenoid(eus), thyroepiglottic(us), and vocal(is). [NIH]

Larynx: An irregularly shaped, musculocartilaginous tubular structure, lined with mucous membrane, located at the top of the trachea and below the root of the tongue and the hyoid bone. It is the essential sphincter guarding the entrance into the trachea and functioning secondarily as the organ of voice. [NIH]

Lesion: An area of abnormal tissue change. [NIH]

Leukemia: Cancer of blood-forming tissue. [NIH]

Levo: It is an experimental treatment for heroin addiction that was developed by German scientists around 1948 as an analgesic. Like methadone, it binds with opioid receptors, but it is longer acting. [NIH]

Levodopa: The naturally occurring form of dopa and the immediate precursor of dopamine. Unlike dopamine itself, it can be taken orally and crosses the blood-brain barrier. It is rapidly taken up by dopaminergic neurons and converted to dopamine. It is used for the treatment of parkinsonism and is usually given with agents that inhibit its conversion to dopamine outside of the central nervous system. [NIH]

Life Expectancy: A figure representing the number of years, based on known statistics, to which any person of a given age may reasonably expect to live. [NIH]

Limbic: Pertaining to a limbus, or margin; forming a border around. [EU]

Limbic System: A set of forebrain structures common to all mammals that is defined functionally and anatomically. It is implicated in the higher integration of visceral, olfactory, and somatic information as well as homeostatic responses including fundamental survival behaviors (feeding, mating, emotion). For most authors, it includes the amygdala, epithalamus, gyrus cinguli, hippocampal formation (see hippocampus), hypothalamus, parahippocampal gyrus, septal nuclei, anterior nuclear group of thalamus, and portions of the basal ganglia. (Parent, Carpenter's Human Neuroanatomy, 9th ed, p744; NeuroNames, http://rprcsgi.rprc.washington.edu/neuronames/index.html (September 2, 1998)). [NIH]

Linkage: The tendency of two or more genes in the same chromosome to remain together from one generation to the next more frequently than expected according to the law of independent assortment. [NIH]

Linkage Disequilibrium: Nonrandom association of linked genes. This is the tendency of the alleles of two separate but already linked loci to be found together more frequently than would be expected by chance alone. [NIH]

Lipid: Fat. [NIH]

Lithium: An element in the alkali metals family. It has the atomic symbol Li, atomic number 3, and atomic weight 6.94. Salts of lithium are used in treating manic-depressive disorders. [NIH]

Liver: A large, glandular organ located in the upper abdomen. The liver cleanses the blood and aids in digestion by secreting bile. [NIH]

Lobe: A portion of an organ such as the liver, lung, breast, or brain. [NIH]

Localization: The process of determining or marking the location or site of a lesion or disease. May also refer to the process of keeping a lesion or disease in a specific location or site. [NIH]

Low Back Pain: Acute or chronic pain in the lumbar or sacral regions, which may be associated with musculo-ligamentous sprains and strains; intervertebral disk displacement; and other conditions. [NIH]

Lumbar: Pertaining to the loins, the part of the back between the thorax and the pelvis. [EU]

Lymph: The almost colorless fluid that travels through the lymphatic system and carries cells that help fight infection and disease. [NIH]

Lymph node: A rounded mass of lymphatic tissue that is surrounded by a capsule of connective tissue. Also known as a lymph gland. Lymph nodes are spread out along lymphatic vessels and contain many lymphocytes, which filter the lymphatic fluid (lymph). [NIH]

Magnetic Resonance Imaging: Non-invasive method of demonstrating internal anatomy based on the principle that atomic nuclei in a strong magnetic field absorb pulses of radiofrequency energy and emit them as radiowaves which can be reconstructed into computerized images. The concept includes proton spin tomographic techniques. [NIH]

Magnetic Resonance Spectroscopy: Spectroscopic method of measuring the magnetic moment of elementary particles such as atomic nuclei, protons or electrons. It is employed in clinical applications such as NMR Tomography (magnetic resonance imaging). [NIH]

Major Histocompatibility Complex: The genetic region which contains the loci of genes which determine the structure of the serologically defined (SD) and lymphocyte-defined (LD) transplantation antigens, genes which control the structure of the immune response-associated (Ia) antigens, the immune response (Ir) genes which control the ability of an animal to respond immunologically to antigenic stimuli, and genes which determine the structure and/or level of the first four components of complement. [NIH]

Manic: Affected with mania. [EU]

Manifest: Being the part or aspect of a phenomenon that is directly observable : concretely expressed in behaviour. [EU]

Medial: Lying near the midsaggital plane of the body; opposed to lateral. [NIH]

Median Nerve: A major nerve of the upper extremity. In humans, the fibers of the median nerve originate in the lower cervical and upper thoracic spinal cord (usually C6 to T1), travel via the brachial plexus, and supply sensory and motor innervation to parts of the forearm and hand. [NIH]

Mediator: An object or substance by which something is mediated, such as (1) a structure of the nervous system that transmits impulses eliciting a specific response; (2) a chemical substance (transmitter substance) that induces activity in an excitable tissue, such as nerve or muscle; or (3) a substance released from cells as the result of the interaction of antigen with antibody or by the action of antigen with a sensitized lymphocyte. [EU]

MEDLINE: An online database of MEDLARS, the computerized bibliographic Medical Literature Analysis and Retrieval System of the National Library of Medicine. [NIH]

Membrane: A very thin layer of tissue that covers a surface. [NIH]

Memory: Complex mental function having four distinct phases: (1) memorizing or learning, (2) retention, (3) recall, and (4) recognition. Clinically, it is usually subdivided into immediate, recent, and remote memory. [NIH]

Menopause: Permanent cessation of menstruation. [NIH]

Mental: Pertaining to the mind; psychic. 2. (L. mentum chin) pertaining to the chin. [EU]

Mercury: A silver metallic element that exists as a liquid at room temperature. It has the atomic symbol Hg (from hydrargyrum, liquid silver), atomic number 80, and atomic weight 200.59. Mercury is used in many industrial applications and its salts have been employed therapeutically as purgatives, antisyphilitics, disinfectants, and astringents. It can be absorbed through the skin and mucous membranes which leads to mercury poisoning. Because of its toxicity, the clinical use of mercury and mercurials is diminishing. [NIH]

Mesolimbic: Inner brain region governing emotion and drives. [NIH]

Methazolamide: A carbonic anhydrase inhibitor that is used as a diuretic and in the treatment of glaucoma. [NIH]

Metoprolol: Adrenergic beta-1-blocking agent with no stimulatory action. It is less bound to plasma albumin than alprenolol and may be useful in angina pectoris, hypertension, or cardiac arrhythmias. [NIH]

MI: Myocardial infarction. Gross necrosis of the myocardium as a result of interruption of the blood supply to the area; it is almost always caused by atherosclerosis of the coronary arteries, upon which coronary thrombosis is usually superimposed. [NIH]

Modification: A change in an organism, or in a process in an organism, that is acquired from its own activity or environment. [NIH]

Molecular: Of, pertaining to, or composed of molecules : a very small mass of matter. [EU]

Molecule: A chemical made up of two or more atoms. The atoms in a molecule can be the same (an oxygen molecule has two oxygen atoms) or different (a water molecule has two hydrogen atoms and one oxygen atom). Biological molecules, such as proteins and DNA, can be made up of many thousands of atoms. [NIH]

Monitor: An apparatus which automatically records such physiological signs as respiration, pulse, and blood pressure in an anesthetized patient or one undergoing surgical or other procedures. [NIH]

Monotherapy: A therapy which uses only one drug. [EU]

Morphological: Relating to the configuration or the structure of live organs. [NIH]

Motility: The ability to move spontaneously. [EU]

Motor Cortex: Area of the frontal lobe concerned with primary motor control. It lies anterior to the central sulcus. [NIH]

Multiple sclerosis: A disorder of the central nervous system marked by weakness, numbness, a loss of muscle coordination, and problems with vision, speech, and bladder control. Multiple sclerosis is thought to be an autoimmune disease in which the body's immune system destroys myelin. Myelin is a substance that contains both protein and fat (lipid) and serves as a nerve insulator and helps in the transmission of nerve signals. [NIH]

Muscimol: Neurotoxic isoxazole isolated from Amanita muscaria and A. phalloides and also obtained by decarboxylation of ibotenic acid. It is a potent agonist at GABA-A receptors and is used mainly as an experimental tool in animal and tissue studies. [NIH]

Muscular Dystrophies: A general term for a group of inherited disorders which are characterized by progressive degeneration of skeletal muscles. [NIH]

Musculature: The muscular apparatus of the body, or of any part of it. [EU]

Myelin: The fatty substance that covers and protects nerves. [NIH]

Myocardial infarction: Gross necrosis of the myocardium as a result of interruption of the blood supply to the area; it is almost always caused by atherosclerosis of the coronary arteries, upon which coronary thrombosis is usually superimposed. [NIH]

Myocardium: The muscle tissue of the heart composed of striated, involuntary muscle known as cardiac muscle. [NIH]

Myoclonus: Involuntary shock-like contractions, irregular in rhythm and amplitude, followed by relaxation, of a muscle or a group of muscles. This condition may be a feature of some central nervous systems diseases (e.g., epilepsy, myoclonic). Nocturnal myoclonus may represent a normal physiologic event or occur as the principal feature of the nocturnal myoclonus syndrome. (From Adams et al., Principles of Neurology, 6th ed, pp102-3). [NIH]

Nausea: An unpleasant sensation in the stomach usually accompanied by the urge to vomit. Common causes are early pregnancy, sea and motion sickness, emotional stress, intense pain, food poisoning, and various enteroviruses. [NIH]

Necrosis: A pathological process caused by the progressive degradative action of enzymes that is generally associated with severe cellular trauma. It is characterized by mitochondrial swelling, nuclear flocculation, uncontrolled cell lysis, and ultimately cell death. [NIH]

Nerve: A cordlike structure of nervous tissue that connects parts of the nervous system with other tissues of the body and conveys nervous impulses to, or away from, these tissues. [NIH]

Nervous System: The entire nerve apparatus composed of the brain, spinal cord, nerves and ganglia. [NIH]

Neural: 1. Pertaining to a nerve or to the nerves. 2. Situated in the region of the spinal axis, as the neutral arch. [EU]

Neural Pathways: Neural tracts connecting one part of the nervous system with another. [NIH]

Neuroanatomy: Study of the anatomy of the nervous system as a specialty or discipline. [NIH]

Neurodegenerative Diseases: Hereditary and sporadic conditions which are characterized by progressive nervous system dysfunction. These disorders are often associated with atrophy of the affected central or peripheral nervous system structures. [NIH]

Neuroleptic: A term coined to refer to the effects on cognition and behaviour of antipsychotic drugs, which produce a state of apathy, lack of initiative, and limited range of emotion and in psychotic patients cause a reduction in confusion and agitation and normalization of psychomotor activity. [EU]

Neurologic: Having to do with nerves or the nervous system. [NIH]

Neuromuscular: Pertaining to muscles and nerves. [EU]

Neuromuscular Junction: The synapse between a neuron and a muscle. [NIH]

Neuronal: Pertaining to a neuron or neurons (= conducting cells of the nervous system). [EU]

Neurons: The basic cellular units of nervous tissue. Each neuron consists of a body, an axon, and dendrites. Their purpose is to receive, conduct, and transmit impulses in the nervous system. [NIH]

Neuropathy: A problem in any part of the nervous system except the brain and spinal cord. Neuropathies can be caused by infection, toxic substances, or disease. [NIH]

Neurosis: Functional derangement due to disorders of the nervous system which does not affect the psychic personality of the patient. [NIH]

Neurotoxicity: The tendency of some treatments to cause damage to the nervous system. [NIH]

Neurotoxin: A substance that is poisonous to nerve tissue. [NIH]

Neurotransmitter: Any of a group of substances that are released on excitation from the axon terminal of a presynaptic neuron of the central or peripheral nervous system and travel across the synaptic cleft to either excite or inhibit the target cell. Among the many substances that have the properties of a neurotransmitter are acetylcholine, norepinephrine, epinephrine, dopamine, glycine, y-aminobutyrate, glutamic acid, substance P, enkephalins, endorphins, and serotonin. [EU]

Niacin: Water-soluble vitamin of the B complex occurring in various animal and plant tissues. Required by the body for the formation of coenzymes NAD and NADP. Has pellagra-curative, vasodilating, and antilipemic properties. [NIH]

Nictitating Membrane: A fold of the mucous membrane of the conjunctiva in many animals. At rest, it is hidden in the medial canthus. It can extend to cover part or all of the cornea to help clean the cornea. [NIH]

Nitrogen: An element with the atomic symbol N, atomic number 7, and atomic weight 14. Nitrogen exists as a diatomic gas and makes up about 78% of the earth's atmosphere by volume. It is a constituent of proteins and nucleic acids and found in all living cells. [NIH]

Norepinephrine: Precursor of epinephrine that is secreted by the adrenal medulla and is a widespread central and autonomic neurotransmitter. Norepinephrine is the principal transmitter of most postganglionic sympathetic fibers and of the diffuse projection system in the brain arising from the locus ceruleus. It is also found in plants and is used pharmacologically as a sympathomimetic. [NIH]

Nuclear: A test of the structure, blood flow, and function of the kidneys. The doctor injects a mildly radioactive solution into an arm vein and uses x-rays to monitor its progress through the kidneys. [NIH]

Nuclei: A body of specialized protoplasm found in nearly all cells and containing the chromosomes. [NIH]

Nucleus: A body of specialized protoplasm found in nearly all cells and containing the chromosomes. [NIH]

Obsessive-Compulsive Disorder: An anxiety disorder characterized by recurrent, persistent obsessions or compulsions. Obsessions are the intrusive ideas, thoughts, or images that are experienced as senseless or repugnant. Compulsions are repetitive and seemingly purposeful behavior which the individual generally recognizes as senseless and from which the individual does not derive pleasure although it may provide a release from tension. [NIH]

Occipital Lobe: Posterior part of the cerebral hemisphere. [NIH]

Occupational Exposure: The exposure to potentially harmful chemical, physical, or biological agents that occurs as a result of one's occupation. [NIH]

Oculi: Globe or ball of the eye. [NIH]

Opacity: Degree of density (area most dense taken for reading). [NIH]

Orbicularis: A thin layer of fibers that originates at the posterior lacrimal crest and passes outward and forward, dividing into two slips which surround the canaliculi. [NIH]

Orthostatic: Pertaining to or caused by standing erect. [EU]

Ossicles: The hammer, anvil and stirrup, the small bones of the middle ear, which transmit the vibrations from the tympanic membrane to the oval window. [NIH]

Oxygenation: The process of supplying, treating, or mixing with oxygen. No:1245 - oxygenation the process of supplying, treating, or mixing with oxygen. [EU]

Palliative: 1. Affording relief, but not cure. 2. An alleviating medicine. [EU]

Palsy: Disease of the peripheral nervous system occurring usually after many years of increased lead absorption. [NIH]

Pancreas: A mixed exocrine and endocrine gland situated transversely across the posterior abdominal wall in the epigastric and hypochondriac regions. The endocrine portion is comprised of the Islets of Langerhans, while the exocrine portion is a compound acinar gland that secretes digestive enzymes. [NIH]

Paralysis: Loss of ability to move all or part of the body. [NIH]

Parkinsonism: A group of neurological disorders characterized by hypokinesia, tremor, and muscular rigidity. [EU]

Paroxysmal: Recurring in paroxysms (= spasms or seizures). [EU]

Pathogenesis: The cellular events and reactions that occur in the development of disease. [NIH]

Pathophysiology: Altered functions in an individual or an organ due to disease. [NIH]

Patient Education: The teaching or training of patients concerning their own health needs. [NIH]

Peripheral Nervous System: The nervous system outside of the brain and spinal cord. The peripheral nervous system has autonomic and somatic divisions. The autonomic nervous system includes the enteric, parasympathetic, and sympathetic subdivisions. The somatic nervous system includes the cranial and spinal nerves and their ganglia and the peripheral sensory receptors. [NIH]

Peripheral Neuropathy: Nerve damage, usually affecting the feet and legs; causing pain, numbness, or a tingling feeling. Also called "somatic neuropathy" or "distal sensory polyneuropathy." [NIH]

Peripheral Vascular Disease: Disease in the large blood vessels of the arms, legs, and feet. People who have had diabetes for a long time may get this because major blood vessels in their arms, legs, and feet are blocked and these limbs do not receive enough blood. The signs of PVD are aching pains in the arms, legs, and feet (especially when walking) and foot sores that heal slowly. Although people with diabetes cannot always avoid PVD, doctors say they have a better chance of avoiding it if they take good care of their feet, do not smoke, and keep both their blood pressure and diabetes under good control. [NIH]

Pesticides: Chemicals used to destroy pests of any sort. The concept includes fungicides (industrial fungicides), insecticides, rodenticides, etc. [NIH]

Pharmacologic: Pertaining to pharmacology or to the properties and reactions of drugs. [EU]

Phenobarbital: A barbituric acid derivative that acts as a nonselective central nervous system depressant. It promotes binding to inhibitory GABA subtype receptors, and modulates chloride currents through receptor channels. It also inhibits glutamate induced depolarizations. [NIH]

Phenotype: The outward appearance of the individual. It is the product of interactions between genes and between the genotype and the environment. This includes the killer phenotype, characteristic of yeasts. [NIH]

Phenoxybenzamine: An alpha-adrenergic antagonist with long duration of action. It has been used to treat hypertension and as a peripheral vasodilator. [NIH]

Phobia: A persistent, irrational, intense fear of a specific object, activity, or situation (the phobic stimulus), fear that is recognized as being excessive or unreasonable by the individual himself. When a phobia is a significant source of distress or interferes with social functioning, it is considered a mental disorder; phobic disorder (or neurosis). In DSM III phobic disorders are subclassified as agoraphobia, social phobias, and simple phobias. Used as a word termination denoting irrational fear of or aversion to the subject indicated by the stem to which it is affixed. [EU]

Phobic Disorders: Anxiety disorders in which the essential feature is persistent and irrational fear of a specific object, activity, or situation that the individual feels compelled to avoid. The individual recognizes the fear as excessive or unreasonable. [NIH]

Phonation: The process of producing vocal sounds by means of vocal cords vibrating in an expiratory blast of air. [NIH]

Physiologic: Having to do with the functions of the body. When used in the phrase "physiologic age," it refers to an age assigned by general health, as opposed to calendar age. [NIH]

Physiology: The science that deals with the life processes and functions of organismus, their cells, tissues, and organs. [NIH]

Pilot study: The initial study examining a new method or treatment. [NIH]

Pitch: The subjective awareness of the frequency or spectral distribution of a sound. [NIH]

Plants: Multicellular, eukaryotic life forms of the kingdom Plantae. They are characterized by a mainly photosynthetic mode of nutrition; essentially unlimited growth at localized regions of cell divisions (meristems); cellulose within cells providing rigidity; the absence of organs of locomotion; absense of nervous and sensory systems; and an alteration of haploid and diploid generations. [NIH]

Plasma: The clear, yellowish, fluid part of the blood that carries the blood cells. The proteins that form blood clots are in plasma. [NIH]

Pneumonia: Inflammation of the lungs. [NIH]

Poisoning: A condition or physical state produced by the ingestion, injection or inhalation of, or exposure to a deleterious agent. [NIH]

Posterior: Situated in back of, or in the back part of, or affecting the back or dorsal surface of the body. In lower animals, it refers to the caudal end of the body. [EU]

Postsynaptic: Nerve potential generated by an inhibitory hyperpolarizing stimulation. [NIH]

Postural: Pertaining to posture or position. [EU]

Practice Guidelines: Directions or principles presenting current or future rules of policy for the health care practitioner to assist him in patient care decisions regarding diagnosis, therapy, or related clinical circumstances. The guidelines may be developed by government agencies at any level, institutions, professional societies, governing boards, or by the convening of expert panels. The guidelines form a basis for the evaluation of all aspects of health care and delivery. [NIH]

Precursor: Something that precedes. In biological processes, a substance from which another, usually more active or mature substance is formed. In clinical medicine, a sign or symptom that heralds another. [EU]

Prefrontal Cortex: The rostral part of the frontal lobe, bounded by the inferior precentral fissure in humans, which receives projection fibers from the mediodorsal nucleus of the thalamus. The prefrontal cortex receives afferent fibers from numerous structures of the diencephalon, mesencephalon, and limbic system as well as cortical afferents of visual, auditory, and somatic origin. [NIH]

Prenatal: Existing or occurring before birth, with reference to the fetus. [EU]

Presynaptic: Situated proximal to a synapse, or occurring before the synapse is crossed. [EU]

Prevalence: The total number of cases of a given disease in a specified population at a designated time. It is differentiated from incidence, which refers to the number of new cases in the population at a given time. [NIH]

Probe: An instrument used in exploring cavities, or in the detection and dilatation of strictures, or in demonstrating the potency of channels; an elongated instrument for exploring or sounding body cavities. [NIH]

Procaine: A local anesthetic of the ester type that has a slow onset and a short duration of action. It is mainly used for infiltration anesthesia, peripheral nerve block, and spinal block. (From Martindale, The Extra Pharmacopoeia, 30th ed, p1016). [NIH]

Progression: Increase in the size of a tumor or spread of cancer in the body. [NIH]

Progressive: Advancing; going forward; going from bad to worse; increasing in scope or severity. [EU]

Projection: A defense mechanism, operating unconsciously, whereby that which is emotionally unacceptable in the self is rejected and attributed (projected) to others. [NIH]

Prophylaxis: An attempt to prevent disease. [NIH]

Propoxur: A carbamate insecticide. [NIH]

Propranolol: A widely used non-cardioselective beta-adrenergic antagonist. Propranolol is used in the treatment or prevention of many disorders including acute myocardial infarction, arrhythmias, angina pectoris, hypertension, hypertensive emergencies, hyperthyroidism, migraine, pheochromocytoma, menopause, and anxiety. [NIH]

Prospective study: An epidemiologic study in which a group of individuals (a cohort), all free of a particular disease and varying in their exposure to a possible risk factor, is followed over a specific amount of time to determine the incidence rates of the disease in the exposed and unexposed groups. [NIH]

Prostate: A gland in males that surrounds the neck of the bladder and the urethra. It secretes a substance that liquifies coagulated semen. It is situated in the pelvic cavity behind the lower part of the pubic symphysis, above the deep layer of the triangular ligament, and rests upon the rectum. [NIH]

Protein S: The vitamin K-dependent cofactor of activated protein C. Together with protein C, it inhibits the action of factors VIIIa and Va. A deficiency in protein S can lead to recurrent venous and arterial thrombosis. [NIH]

Proteins: Polymers of amino acids linked by peptide bonds. The specific sequence of amino acids determines the shape and function of the protein. [NIH]

Protocol: The detailed plan for a clinical trial that states the trial's rationale, purpose, drug or vaccine dosages, length of study, routes of administration, who may participate, and other aspects of trial design. [NIH]

Protons: Stable elementary particles having the smallest known positive charge, found in the nuclei of all elements. The proton mass is less than that of a neutron. A proton is the nucleus of the light hydrogen atom, i.e., the hydrogen ion. [NIH]

Psychiatric: Pertaining to or within the purview of psychiatry. [EU]

Psychiatry: The medical science that deals with the origin, diagnosis, prevention, and treatment of mental disorders. [NIH]

Psychic: Pertaining to the psyche or to the mind; mental. [EU]

Psychosis: A mental disorder characterized by gross impairment in reality testing as evidenced by delusions, hallucinations, markedly incoherent speech, or disorganized and agitated behaviour without apparent awareness on the part of the patient of the incomprehensibility of his behaviour; the term is also used in a more general sense to refer to mental disorders in which mental functioning is sufficiently impaired as to interfere grossly with the patient's capacity to meet the ordinary demands of life. Historically, the term has been applied to many conditions, e.g. manic-depressive psychosis, that were first described in psychotic patients, although many patients with the disorder are not judged psychotic. [EU]

Public Policy: A course or method of action selected, usually by a government, from among alternatives to guide and determine present and future decisions. [NIH]

Pulse: The rhythmical expansion and contraction of an artery produced by waves of pressure caused by the ejection of blood from the left ventricle of the heart as it contracts. [NIH]

Quality of Life: A generic concept reflecting concern with the modification and enhancement of life attributes, e.g., physical, political, moral and social environment. [NIH]

Race: A population within a species which exhibits general similarities within itself, but is both discontinuous and distinct from other populations of that species, though not sufficiently so as to achieve the status of a taxon. [NIH]

Racemic: Optically inactive but resolvable in the way of all racemic compounds. [NIH]

Radiation: Emission or propagation of electromagnetic energy (waves/rays), or the waves/rays themselves; a stream of electromagnetic particles (electrons, neutrons, protons, alpha particles) or a mixture of these. The most common source is the sun. [NIH]

Radioactive: Giving off radiation. [NIH]

Randomized: Describes an experiment or clinical trial in which animal or human subjects are assigned by chance to separate groups that compare different treatments. [NIH]

Receptor: A molecule inside or on the surface of a cell that binds to a specific substance and causes a specific physiologic effect in the cell. [NIH]

Receptors, Serotonin: Cell-surface proteins that bind serotonin and trigger intracellular changes which influence the behavior of cells. Several types of serotonin receptors have been recognized which differ in their pharmacology, molecular biology, and mode of action. [NIH]

Recombination: The formation of new combinations of genes as a result of segregation in crosses between genetically different parents; also the rearrangement of linked genes due to crossing-over. [NIH]

Refer: To send or direct for treatment, aid, information, de decision. [NIH]

Reflex: An involuntary movement or exercise of function in a part, excited in response to a stimulus applied to the periphery and transmitted to the brain or spinal cord. [NIH]

Refraction: A test to determine the best eyeglasses or contact lenses to correct a refractive error (myopia, hyperopia, or astigmatism). [NIH]

Refractory: Not readily yielding to treatment. [EU]

Regimen: A treatment plan that specifies the dosage, the schedule, and the duration of treatment. [NIH]

Reliability: Used technically, in a statistical sense, of consistency of a test with itself, i. e. the extent to which we can assume that it will yield the same result if repeated a second time. [NIH]

Restless legs: Legs characterized by or showing inability to remain at rest. [EU]

Retroviral vector: RNA from a virus that is used to insert genetic material into cells. [NIH]

Risk factor: A habit, trait, condition, or genetic alteration that increases a person's chance of developing a disease. [NIH]

Sclerosis: A pathological process consisting of hardening or fibrosis of an anatomical structure, often a vessel or a nerve. [NIH]

Scoliosis: A lateral curvature of the spine. [NIH]

Screening: Checking for disease when there are no symptoms. [NIH]

Secretory: Secreting; relating to or influencing secretion or the secretions. [NIH]

Sedative: 1. Allaying activity and excitement. 2. An agent that allays excitement. [EU]

Seizures: Clinical or subclinical disturbances of cortical function due to a sudden, abnormal, excessive, and disorganized discharge of brain cells. Clinical manifestations include abnormal motor, sensory and psychic phenomena. Recurrent seizures are usually referred to as epilepsy or "seizure disorder." [NIH]

Self Care: Performance of activities or tasks traditionally performed by professional health care providers. The concept includes care of oneself or one's family and friends. [NIH]

Senile: Relating or belonging to old age; characteristic of old age; resulting from infirmity of old age. [NIH]

Sensor: A device designed to respond to physical stimuli such as temperature, light, magnetism or movement and transmit resulting impulses for interpretation, recording, movement, or operating control. [NIH]

Septal: An abscess occurring at the root of the tooth on the proximal surface. [NIH]

Septum: A dividing wall or partition; a general term for such a structure. The term is often used alone to refer to the septal area or to the septum pellucidum. [EU]

Septum Pellucidum: A triangular double membrane separating the anterior horns of the lateral ventricles of the brain. It is situated in the median plane and bounded by the corpus callosum and the body and columns of the fornix. [NIH]

Sequencing: The determination of the order of nucleotides in a DNA or RNA chain. [NIH]

Serotonin: A biochemical messenger and regulator, synthesized from the essential amino acid L-tryptophan. In humans it is found primarily in the central nervous system, gastrointestinal tract, and blood platelets. Serotonin mediates several important physiological functions including neurotransmission, gastrointestinal motility, hemostasis, and cardiovascular integrity. Multiple receptor families (receptors, serotonin) explain the broad physiological actions and distribution of this biochemical mediator. [NIH]

Shock: The general bodily disturbance following a severe injury; an emotional or moral upset occasioned by some disturbing or unexpected experience; disruption of the circulation, which can upset all body functions: sometimes referred to as circulatory shock. [NIH]

Side effect: A consequence other than the one(s) for which an agent or measure is used, as the adverse effects produced by a drug, especially on a tissue or organ system other than the one sought to be benefited by its administration. [EU]

Skeletal: Having to do with the skeleton (boney part of the body). [NIH]

Skull: The skeleton of the head including the bones of the face and the bones enclosing the brain. [NIH]

Small intestine: The part of the digestive tract that is located between the stomach and the large intestine. [NIH]

Smooth muscle: Muscle that performs automatic tasks, such as constricting blood vessels. [NIH]

Social Environment: The aggregate of social and cultural institutions, forms, patterns, and processes that influence the life of an individual or community. [NIH]

Solvent: 1. Dissolving; effecting a solution. 2. A liquid that dissolves or that is capable of dissolving; the component of a solution that is present in greater amount. [EU]

Somatic: 1. Pertaining to or characteristic of the soma or body. 2. Pertaining to the body wall in contrast to the viscera. [EU]

Sotalol: An adrenergic beta-antagonist that is used in the treatment of life-threatening arrhythmias. [NIH]

Sound wave: An alteration of properties of an elastic medium, such as pressure, particle displacement, or density, that propagates through the medium, or a superposition of such alterations. [NIH]

Spasm: An involuntary contraction of a muscle or group of muscles. Spasms may involve skeletal muscle or smooth muscle. [NIH]

Spasmodic: Of the nature of a spasm. [EU]

Specialist: In medicine, one who concentrates on 1 special branch of medical science. [NIH]

Species: A taxonomic category subordinate to a genus (or subgenus) and superior to a subspecies or variety, composed of individuals possessing common characters distinguishing them from other categories of individuals of the same taxonomic level. In taxonomic nomenclature, species are designated by the genus name followed by a Latin or Latinized adjective or noun. [EU]

Spectroscopic: The recognition of elements through their emission spectra. [NIH]

Spectrum: A charted band of wavelengths of electromagnetic vibrations obtained by refraction and diffraction. By extension, a measurable range of activity, such as the range of bacteria affected by an antibiotic (antibacterial s.) or the complete range of manifestations of a disease. [EU]

Sperm: The fecundating fluid of the male. [NIH]

Spinal cord: The main trunk or bundle of nerves running down the spine through holes in the spinal bone (the vertebrae) from the brain to the level of the lower back. [NIH]

Spinal Nerves: The 31 paired peripheral nerves formed by the union of the dorsal and ventral spinal roots from each spinal cord segment. The spinal nerve plexuses and the spinal roots are also included. [NIH]

Sporadic: Neither endemic nor epidemic; occurring occasionally in a random or isolated manner. [EU]

Sprains and Strains: A collective term for muscle and ligament injuries without dislocation or fracture. A sprain is a joint injury in which some of the fibers of a supporting ligament are ruptured but the continuity of the ligament remains intact. A strain is an overstretching or overexertion of some part of the musculature. [NIH]

Stimulant: 1. Producing stimulation; especially producing stimulation by causing tension on muscle fibre through the nervous tissue. 2. An agent or remedy that produces stimulation. [EU]

Stimulus: That which can elicit or evoke action (response) in a muscle, nerve, gland or other excitable issue, or cause an augmenting action upon any function or metabolic process. [NIH]

Stomach: An organ of digestion situated in the left upper quadrant of the abdomen between the termination of the esophagus and the beginning of the duodenum. [NIH]

Strabismus: Deviation of the eye which the patient cannot overcome. The visual axes assume a position relative to each other different from that required by the physiological conditions. The various forms of strabismus are spoken of as tropias, their direction being indicated by the appropriate prefix, as cyclo tropia, esotropia, exotropia, hypertropia, and hypotropia. Called also cast, heterotropia, manifest deviation, and squint. [EU]

Stress: Forcibly exerted influence; pressure. Any condition or situation that causes strain or tension. Stress may be either physical or psychologic, or both. [NIH]

Stroke: Sudden loss of function of part of the brain because of loss of blood flow. Stroke may be caused by a clot (thrombosis) or rupture (hemorrhage) of a blood vessel to the brain. [NIH]

Subclinical: Without clinical manifestations; said of the early stage(s) of an infection or other disease or abnormality before symptoms and signs become apparent or detectable by clinical examination or laboratory tests, or of a very mild form of an infection or other disease or abnormality. [EU]

Sympathomimetic: 1. Mimicking the effects of impulses conveyed by adrenergic postganglionic fibres of the sympathetic nervous system. 2. An agent that produces effects similar to those of impulses conveyed by adrenergic postganglionic fibres of the sympathetic nervous system. Called also adrenergic. [EU]

Symptomatic: Having to do with symptoms, which are signs of a condition or disease. [NIH]

Symptomatic treatment: Therapy that eases symptoms without addressing the cause of disease. [NIH]

Synapse: The region where the processes of two neurons come into close contiguity, and the nervous impulse passes from one to the other; the fibers of the two are intermeshed, but, according to the general view, there is no direct contiguity. [NIH]

Synaptic: Pertaining to or affecting a synapse (= site of functional apposition between neurons, at which an impulse is transmitted from one neuron to another by electrical or chemical means); pertaining to synapsis (= pairing off in point-for-point association of homologous chromosomes from the male and female pronuclei during the early prophase of meiosis). [EU]

Synaptic Vesicles: Membrane-bound compartments which contain transmitter molecules. Synaptic vesicles are concentrated at presynaptic terminals. They actively sequester transmitter molecules from the cytoplasm. In at least some synapses, transmitter release occurs by fusion of these vesicles with the presynaptic membrane, followed by exocytosis of their contents. [NIH]

Synchrony: The normal physiologic sequencing of atrial and ventricular activation and contraction. [NIH]

Systemic: Affecting the entire body. [NIH]

Systemic disease: Disease that affects the whole body. [NIH]

Tardive: Marked by lateness, late; said of a disease in which the characteristic lesion is late in appearing. [EU]

Telecommunications: Transmission of information over distances via electronic means. [NIH]

Telencephalon: Paired anteriolateral evaginations of the prosencephalon plus the lamina terminalis. The cerebral hemispheres are derived from it. Many authors consider cerebrum a synonymous term to telencephalon, though a minority include diencephalon as part of the cerebrum (Anthoney, 1994). [NIH]

Temporal: One of the two irregular bones forming part of the lateral surfaces and base of the skull, and containing the organs of hearing. [NIH]

Temporal Lobe: Lower lateral part of the cerebral hemisphere. [NIH]

Tendon: A discrete band of connective tissue mainly composed of parallel bundles of collagenous fibers by which muscles are attached, or two muscles bellies joined. [NIH]

Thalamic: Cell that reaches the lateral nucleus of amygdala. [NIH]

Thalamus: Paired bodies containing mostly gray substance and forming part of the lateral wall of the third ventricle of the brain. The thalamus represents the major portion of the diencephalon and is commonly divided into cellular aggregates known as nuclear groups. [NIH]

Therapeutics: The branch of medicine which is concerned with the treatment of diseases, palliative or curative. [NIH]

Thoracic: Having to do with the chest. [NIH]

Threshold: For a specified sensory modality (e. g. light, sound, vibration), the lowest level (absolute threshold) or smallest difference (difference threshold, difference limen) or intensity of the stimulus discernible in prescribed conditions of stimulation. [NIH]

Thrombosis: The formation or presence of a blood clot inside a blood vessel. [NIH]

Thrombus: An aggregation of blood factors, primarily platelets and fibrin with entrapment of cellular elements, frequently causing vascular obstruction at the point of its formation.

Some authorities thus differentiate thrombus formation from simple coagulation or clot formation. [EU]

Thyroid: A gland located near the windpipe (trachea) that produces thyroid hormone, which helps regulate growth and metabolism. [NIH]

Tissue: A group or layer of cells that are alike in type and work together to perform a specific function. [NIH]

Tolerance: 1. The ability to endure unusually large doses of a drug or toxin. 2. Acquired drug tolerance; a decreasing response to repeated constant doses of a drug or the need for increasing doses to maintain a constant response. [EU]

Tomography: Imaging methods that result in sharp images of objects located on a chosen plane and blurred images located above or below the plane. [NIH]

Tonic: 1. Producing and restoring the normal tone. 2. Characterized by continuous tension. 3. A term formerly used for a class of medicinal preparations believed to have the power of restoring normal tone to tissue. [EU]

Topical: On the surface of the body. [NIH]

Torsion: A twisting or rotation of a bodily part or member on its axis. [NIH]

Torticollis: Wryneck; a contracted state of the cervical muscles, producing twisting of the neck and an unnatural position of the head. [EU]

Toxic: Having to do with poison or something harmful to the body. Toxic substances usually cause unwanted side effects. [NIH]

Toxicity: The quality of being poisonous, especially the degree of virulence of a toxic microbe or of a poison. [EU]

Toxicology: The science concerned with the detection, chemical composition, and pharmacologic action of toxic substances or poisons and the treatment and prevention of toxic manifestations. [NIH]

Toxin: A poison; frequently used to refer specifically to a protein produced by some higher plants, certain animals, and pathogenic bacteria, which is highly toxic for other living organisms. Such substances are differentiated from the simple chemical poisons and the vegetable alkaloids by their high molecular weight and antigenicity. [EU]

Trachea: The cartilaginous and membranous tube descending from the larynx and branching into the right and left main bronchi. [NIH]

Transcutaneous: Transdermal. [EU]

Transfection: The uptake of naked or purified DNA into cells, usually eukaryotic. It is analogous to bacterial transformation. [NIH]

Transmitter: A chemical substance which effects the passage of nerve impulses from one cell to the other at the synapse. [NIH]

Tremor: Cyclical movement of a body part that can represent either a physiologic process or a manifestation of disease. Intention or action tremor, a common manifestation of cerebellar diseases, is aggravated by movement. In contrast, resting tremor is maximal when there is no attempt at voluntary movement, and occurs as a relatively frequent manifestation of Parkinson disease. [NIH]

Trigger zone: Dolorogenic zone (= producing or causing pain). [EU]

Tryptophan: An essential amino acid that is necessary for normal growth in infants and for nitrogen balance in adults. It is a precursor serotonin and niacin. [NIH]

Tuberculosis: Any of the infectious diseases of man and other animals caused by species of

Mycobacterium. [NIH]

Tuberculostatic: Inhibiting the growth of Mycobacterium tuberculosis. [EU]

Tumor marker: A substance sometimes found in an increased amount in the blood, other body fluids, or tissues and which may mean that a certain type of cancer is in the body. Examples of tumor markers include CA 125 (ovarian cancer), CA 15-3 (breast cancer), CEA (ovarian, lung, breast, pancreas, and gastrointestinal tract cancers), and PSA (prostate cancer). Also called biomarker. [NIH]

Uterus: The small, hollow, pear-shaped organ in a woman's pelvis. This is the organ in which a fetus develops. Also called the womb. [NIH]

Vascular: Pertaining to blood vessels or indicative of a copious blood supply. [EU]

Vasodilator: An agent that widens blood vessels. [NIH]

VE: The total volume of gas either inspired or expired in one minute. [NIH]

Vein: Vessel-carrying blood from various parts of the body to the heart. [NIH]

Venter: Belly. [NIH]

Ventral: 1. Pertaining to the belly or to any venter. 2. Denoting a position more toward the belly surface than some other object of reference; same as anterior in human anatomy. [EU]

Ventricle: One of the two pumping chambers of the heart. The right ventricle receives oxygen-poor blood from the right atrium and pumps it to the lungs through the pulmonary artery. The left ventricle receives oxygen-rich blood from the left atrium and pumps it to the body through the aorta. [NIH]

Ventricular: Pertaining to a ventricle. [EU]

Venules: The minute vessels that collect blood from the capillary plexuses and join together to form veins. [NIH]

Vertebrae: A bony unit of the segmented spinal column. [NIH]

Vertigo: An illusion of movement; a sensation as if the external world were revolving around the patient (objective vertigo) or as if he himself were revolving in space (subjective vertigo). The term is sometimes erroneously used to mean any form of dizziness. [EU]

Vestibular: Pertaining to or toward a vestibule. In dental anatomy, used to refer to the tooth surface directed toward the vestibule of the mouth. [EU]

Vestibule: A small, oval, bony chamber of the labyrinth. The vestibule contains the utricle and saccule, organs which are part of the balancing apparatus of the ear. [NIH]

Veterinary Medicine: The medical science concerned with the prevention, diagnosis, and treatment of diseases in animals. [NIH]

Vivo: Outside of or removed from the body of a living organism. [NIH]

Vocal cord: The vocal folds of the larynx. [NIH]

Voice Disorders: Disorders of voice pitch, loudness, or quality. Dysphonia refers to impaired utterance of sounds by the vocal folds. [NIH]

Volition: Voluntary activity without external compulsion. [NIH]

Windpipe: A rigid tube, 10 cm long, extending from the cricoid cartilage to the upper border of the fifth thoracic vertebra. [NIH]

Xenograft: The cells of one species transplanted to another species. [NIH]

X-ray: High-energy radiation used in low doses to diagnose diseases and in high doses to treat cancer. [NIH]

Yeasts: A general term for single-celled rounded fungi that reproduce by budding. Brewers' and bakers' yeasts are Saccharomyces cerevisiae; therapeutic dried yeast is dried yeast. [NIH]

INDEX

LaVergne, TN USA
22 November 2009

164934LV00001B/47/A